MW01152286

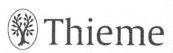

Wide Awake Hand Surgery

Edited by

Donald H. Lalonde, HonsBSc, MD, MSc, FRCSC
Professor, Division of Plastic
and Reconstructive Surgery, Department
of Surgery, Dalhousie University,
Saint John, New Brunswick, Canada

Thieme
New York · Stuttgart · Delhi · Rio de Janeiro

Thieme Medical Publishers, Inc.
333 Seventh Ave.
New York, NY 10001

© 2016 by Thieme Medical Publishers, Inc.

No claim to original U.S. Government works

Printed in the United States of America

International Standard Book Number-13: 978-1-62623-662-2

This book contains information obtained from authentic and highly regarded sources. While all reasonable efforts have been made to publish reliable data and information, neither the author[s] nor the publisher canaccept any legal responsibility or liability for any errors or omissions that may be made. The publishers wish tomake clear that any views or opinions expressed in this book by individual editors, authors or contributors arepersonal to them and do not necessarily reflect the views/opinions of the publishers. The information or guidancecontained in this book is intended for use by medical, scientific or health-care professionals and is providedstrictly as a supplement to the medical or other professional's own judgement, their knowledge of the patient'smedical history, relevant manufacturer's instructions and the appropriate best practice guidelines. Because ofthe rapid advances in medical science, any information or advice on dosages, procedures or diagnoses shouldbe independently verified. The reader is strongly urged to consult the relevant national drug formulary and thedrug companies' and device or material manufacturers' printed instructions, and their websites, before administeringor utilizing any of the drugs, devices or materials mentioned in this book. This book does not indicate whether a particular treatment is appropriate or suitable for a particular individual. Ultimately it is the soleesponsibility of the medical professional to make his or her own professional judgements, so as to advise and treat patients appropriately. The authors and publishers have also attempted to trace the copyright holders of all material reproduced in this publication and apologize to copyright holders if permission to publish in this form has not been obtained. If any copyright material has not been acknowledged please write and let us know
so we may rectify in any future reprint.

Except as permitted under U.S. Copyright Law, no part of this book may be reprinted, reproduced, transmitted, or utilized in any form by any electronic, mechanical, or other means, now known or hereafter invented, including photocopying, microfilming, and recording, or in any information storage or retrieval system, without written permission from the publishers.

For permission to photocopy or use material electronically from this work, please access www.copyright. com (http://www.copyright.com/) or contact the Copyright Clearance Center, Inc. (CCC), 222 Rosewood Drive, Danvers, MA 01923, 978-750-8400. CCC is a not-for-profit organization that provides licenses and registration for a variety of users. For organizations that have been granted a photocopy license by the CCC, a separate system of payment has been arranged.

Trademark Notice: Product or corporate names may be trademarks or registered trademarks, and are used only for identification and explanation without intent to   infringe.

Orders may be sent to: Thieme Publishers New York
333 Seventh Avenue, New York, NY 10001 USA
+1 800 782 3488, customerservice@thieme.com

Thieme Publishers Stuttgart
Rüdigerstrasse 14, 70469 Stuttgart, Germany
+49 [0]711 8931 421, customerservice@thieme.de

Thieme Publishers Delhi
A-12, Second Floor, Sector-2, Noida-201301
Uttar Pradesh, India
+91 120 45 566 00, customerservice@thieme.in

Thieme Publishers Rio de Janeiro, Thieme Publicações Ltda.
Edifício Rodolpho de Paoli, 25º andar
Av. Nilo Peçanha, 50 – Sala 2508,
Rio de Janeiro 20020-906 Brasil
+55 21 3172-2297 / +55 21 3172-1896

www.Thieme.com

CONTRIBUTORS

Julie E. Adams, MD
Associate Professor of Orthopedic Surgery, Mayo Clinic, Rochester, Minnesota

Peter C. Amadio, MD
Lloyd A. and Barbara A. Amundson Professor of Orthopedic Surgery, Mayo Clinic, Rochester, Minnesota

Mark E. Baratz, MD
Clinical Professor and Vice Chairman, Department of Orthopaedics, University of Pittsburgh Medical Center, Pittsburgh, Pennsylvania

Geoff Cook, MD, FRCSC
Assistant Professor, Division of Plastic and Reconstructive Surgery, Department of Surgery, Dalhousie University, Saint John, New Brunswick, Canada

Günter Germann, MD, PhD
Professor of Plastic Surgery–Hand Surgery, University of Heidelberg; Founder and Medical Director, Ethianum Clinic for Plastic, Reconstructive and Aesthetic Surgery, Heidelberg, Baden-Württemberg, Germany

Andrew W. Gurman, MD
Altoona Hand and Wrist Surgery, Altoona, Pennsylvania

Elisabet Hagert, MD, PhD
Associate Professor, Department of Clinical Science and Education, Karolinska Institutet; Chief of Hand Surgery, Hand and Foot Surgery Center, Stockholm, Sweden

Amanda Higgins, BSc, OT
Rothesay, New Brunswick, Canada

Nikolas Alan Jagodzinski, MBChB, FHEM, FRCS (Tr & Orth)
Department of Orthoplastics Hand Surgery, Oxford University Hospitals NHS Trust, Oxford, United Kingdom

Susan Kean, PT, CHT
Rothesay, New Brunswick, Canada

Carolyn L. Kerrigan, MD, MHCDS
Professor, Department of Surgery, Dartmouth-Hitchcock Medical Center, Lebanon, New Hampshire

Donald H. Lalonde, HonsBSc, MD, MSc, FRCSC
Professor, Division of Plastic and Reconstructive Surgery, Department of Surgery, Dalhousie University, Saint John, New Brunswick, Canada

Duncan McGrouther, MD
Senior Consultant Hand Surgeon, Department of Hand Surgery, Singapore General Hospital, Singapore

Michael W. Neumeister, MD, FRCSC, FACS
Professor and Chairman, Department of Surgery, Southern Illinois University of Medicine, Springfield, Illinois

Alistair Phillips, MD
Department of Trauma and Orthopaedic Surgery, University Hospital Southampton NHS Foundation Trust, Southampton, Hampshire, United Kingdom

Michael Sauerbier, MD, PhD
Professor, Department of Plastic, Hand and Reconstructive Surgery, BG Trauma Center Frankfort am Main, Academic Hospital of Goethe University, Frankfurt am Main, Germany

Robert M. Szabo, MD, MPH
Professor of Orthopaedics and Plastic Surgery; Chief of Hand, Microvascular and Upper Extremity Surgery, Department of Orthopaedics, University of California, Davis, Sacramento, California

Jin Bo Tang, MD
Professor and Chair, Department of Hand Surgery, Affiliated Hospital of Nantong University, Nantong, Jiangsu, China

Robert E. Van Demark, Jr., MD, FACS
Section Head and Clinical Professor, Department of Orthopedic Surgery, Sanford School of Medicine, The University of South Dakota, Vermillion, South Dakota

Jason Wong, MBChB, FHEA, PhD, FRCS(Plast)
Honorary Senior Clinical Lecturer and Consultant in Plastic Surgery, University Hospital of South Manchester, Manchester, United Kingdom

Shu Guo Xing, MD
Attending Surgeon, Department of Hand Surgery, Affiliated Hospital of Nantong University, Nantong, Jiangsu, China

Jeffrey Yao, MD
Associate Professor, Department of Orthopaedic Surgery, Stanford University Medical Center, Palo Alto, California

PREFACE

It has been my great privilege to share in the development of this exciting new way of performing hand surgery with many of my colleagues in Canada and around the world. It is an even greater thrill to be able to convey the elements of this technique to the rest of the world's hand surgeons with this first "recipe cookbook" on *How To Do It*.

The goal of this book is that any hand surgeon can pick it up and be able to perform most operations in hand surgery with the wide awake approach in very little time and with very little patient discomfort. To accompany the brief bullet-style text, there are more than 150 short instructional video clips, and the whole package is also available as an e-book for use on the go.

All author royalties from the sale of this book will go to the Lean and Green project of the American Association for Hand Surgery, which promotes less wasted cost and garbage production in hand surgery.

Donald H. Lalonde
dlalonde@drlalonde.ca

ACKNOWLEDGMENTS

I owe the greatest debt of gratitude to my wife, Jan. Her never-ending support and encouragement has made this book possible, with all the research that went into the work behind it.

I also want to thank the many hand surgeons, therapists, and patients in Saint John, New Brunswick, Canada, and the rest of the world who contributed their thoughts and experience into the development of this technique.

CONTENTS

PART I ATLAS OF TUMESCENT LOCAL ANESTHESIA
WITH FOREARM, WRIST, HAND, AND FINGER
INJECTIONS

1 Atlas of Images of Local Anesthetic Diffusion Anatomy 3
Donald H. Lalonde

PART II GENERAL PRINCIPLES OF WIDE AWAKE
HAND SURGERY

2 What Is Wide Awake Hand Surgery? 17
Alistair Phillips, Nik Jagodzinski, Donald H. Lalonde

▶ Video Clips 2-1, 2-2

3 Safe Epinephrine in the Finger Means No Tourniquet 23
Donald H. Lalonde

▶ Video Clips 3-1, 3-2

4 Tumescent Local Anesthesia 29
Donald H. Lalonde, Alistair Phillips, Duncan McGrouther

▶ Video Clip 4-1

5 How to Inject Local Anesthetic With Minimal Pain 37
Donald H. Lalonde, Nik Jagodzinski, Alistair Phillips

▶ Video Clips 5-1, 5-2, 5-3, 5-4, 5-5, 5-6

6 Dealing With Systemic Adverse Reactions to Lidocaine
and Epinephrine 49
Donald H. Lalonde

▶ Video Clips 6-1, 6-2

7 Tips on Talking to Your Patients About WALANT **55**
Nik Jagodzinski, Alistair Phillips, Donald H. Lalonde

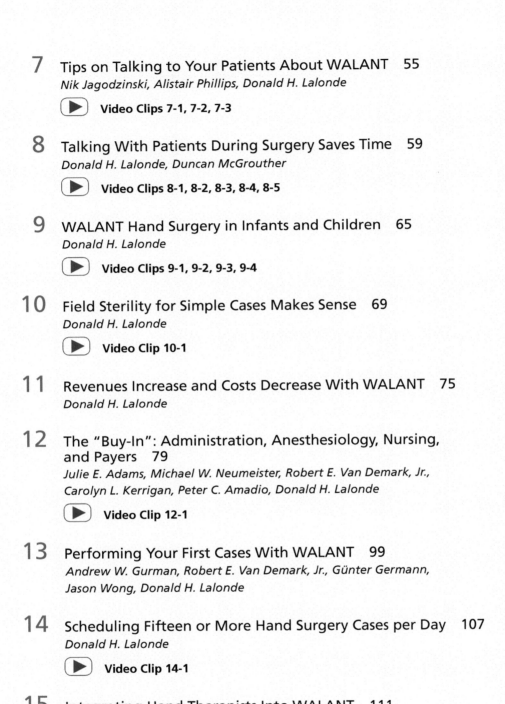 **Video Clips 7-1, 7-2, 7-3**

8 Talking With Patients During Surgery Saves Time **59**
Donald H. Lalonde, Duncan McGrouther

Video Clips 8-1, 8-2, 8-3, 8-4, 8-5

9 WALANT Hand Surgery in Infants and Children **65**
Donald H. Lalonde

Video Clips 9-1, 9-2, 9-3, 9-4

10 Field Sterility for Simple Cases Makes Sense **69**
Donald H. Lalonde

Video Clip 10-1

11 Revenues Increase and Costs Decrease With WALANT **75**
Donald H. Lalonde

12 The "Buy-In": Administration, Anesthesiology, Nursing, and Payers **79**
Julie E. Adams, Michael W. Neumeister, Robert E. Van Demark, Jr., Carolyn L. Kerrigan, Peter C. Amadio, Donald H. Lalonde

Video Clip 12-1

13 Performing Your First Cases With WALANT **99**
Andrew W. Gurman, Robert E. Van Demark, Jr., Günter Germann, Jason Wong, Donald H. Lalonde

14 Scheduling Fifteen or More Hand Surgery Cases per Day **107**
Donald H. Lalonde

Video Clip 14-1

15 Integrating Hand Therapists Into WALANT **111**
Susan Kean, Amanda Higgins, Donald H. Lalonde

Video Clips 15-1, 15-2, 15-3, 15-4, 15-5, 15-6, 15-7, 15-8

16 Minor Procedure Room Setup 117
Donald H. Lalonde, Geoff Cook

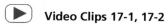 Video Clips 16-1, 16-2, 16-3

PART III SPECIFIC DETAILS OF HOW TO PERFORM WIDE AWAKE HAND SURGERY FOR COMMON OPERATIONS

SECTION A AMPUTATION

17 Finger and Ray Amputation 125
Donald H. Lalonde

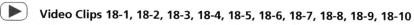 Video Clips 17-1, 17-2

SECTION B NERVE DECOMPRESSION

18 Carpal Tunnel Decompression of the Median Nerve 129
Carolyn L. Kerrigan, Donald H. Lalonde, Shu Guo Xing, Jin Bo Tang

Video Clips 18-1, 18-2, 18-3, 18-4, 18-5, 18-6, 18-7, 18-8, 18-9, 18-10

19 Cubital Tunnel Decompression of the Ulnar Nerve 137
Donald H. Lalonde, Alistair Phillips

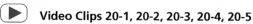 Video Clips 19-1, 19-2, 19-3, 19-4, 19-5, 19-6, 19-7

20 Lacertus Syndrome: Median Nerve Release at the Elbow 141
Elisabet Hagert, Donald H. Lalonde

Video Clips 20-1, 20-2, 20-3, 20-4, 20-5

SECTION C TENDON DECOMPRESSION

21 Trigger Finger 145
Donald H. Lalonde

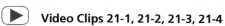 Video Clips 21-1, 21-2, 21-3, 21-4

22 De Quervain Release 149
Donald H. Lalonde, Alistair Phillips

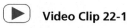 Video Clip 22-1

SECTION D DUPUYTREN'S CONTRACTURE AND SOFT TISSUE EXCISION

23 Dupuytren's Contracture 151
Duncan McGrouther, Jason Wong, Donald H. Lalonde

▶ Video Clips 23-1, 23-2

24 Flexor Sheath Ganglion 155
Donald H. Lalonde

25 Small Soft Tissue Operations 157
Donald H. Lalonde, Jason Wong, Shu Guo Xing, Jin Bo Tang

▶ Video Clips 25-1, 25-2

SECTION E ARTHRITIS SURGERY

26 Arthroplasty of the Proximal Interphalangeal Joint 161
Donald H. Lalonde

▶ Video Clip 26-1

27 Trapeziectomy With or Without Ligament Reconstruction for Thumb Basal Joint Arthritis 165
Donald H. Lalonde, Peter C. Amadio, Geoff Cook

▶ Video Clips 27-1, 27-2, 27-3, 27-4, 27-5, 27-6, 27-7, 27-8

28 Thumb Metacarpophalangeal Joint Fusion and Ulnar Collateral Ligament Repair 171
Donald H. Lalonde

▶ Video Clips 28-1, 28-2, 28-3

29 Proximal Interphalangeal Joint Fusion 175
Donald H. Lalonde

SECTION F WRIST SURGERY

30 Wrist Arthroscopy 179
Elisabet Hagert, Donald H. Lalonde

▶ Video Clip 30-1

31 Open Triangular Fibrocartilage Complex Repair 183
Elisabet Hagert, Donald H. Lalonde

▶ Video Clip 31-1

SECTION G   LACERATED TENDONS AND TENOLYSIS

32 Flexor Tendon Repair of the Finger 187
Jin Bo Tang, Shu Guo Xing, Jason Wong, Jeffrey Yao, Donald H. Lalonde

▶ Video Clips 32-1, 32-2, 32-3, 32-4, 32-5, 32-6, 32-7, 32-8, 32-9, 32-10, 32-11, 32-12, 32-13, 32-14, 32-15, 32-16, 32-17, 32-18

33 Flexor Tendon Repair of the Hand 199
Donald H. Lalonde

34 Flexor Tendon Repair of the Forearm 205
Donald H. Lalonde

▶ Video Clip 34-1

35 Extensor Tendon Repair of the Finger 209
Donald H. Lalonde

▶ Video Clips 35-1, 35-2, 35-3, 35-4, 35-5

36 Extensor Tendon Repair of the Hand 213
Donald H. Lalonde, Geoff Cook

▶ Video Clips 36-1, 36-2

37 Extensor Tendon Repair of the Forearm 217
Donald H. Lalonde

▶ Video Clip 37-1

38 Tenolysis 221
Jason Wong, Michael Sauerbier, Peter C. Amadio, Donald H. Lalonde

▶ Video Clips 38-1, 38-2, 38-3, 38-4, 38-5

SECTION H   TENDON TRANSFERS

39 Tendon Transfers   227
Donald H. Lalonde, Robert M. Szabo, Mark E. Baratz

▶ **Video Clips 39-1, 39-2, 39-3, 39-4, 39-5, 39-6, 39-7, 39-8**

SECTION I   LACERATED NERVES

40 Lacerated Nerves   233
Donald H. Lalonde

▶ **Video Clip 40-1**

SECTION J   FRACTURES

41 Finger Fractures   237
Donald H. Lalonde

▶ **Video Clips 41-1, 41-2, 41-3, 41-4, 41-5, 41-6, 41-7, 41-8, 41-9, 41-10**

42 Reduction and Internal Fixation of Metacarpal Fractures   243
Shu Guo Xing, Jin Bo Tang, Donald H. Lalonde

▶ **Video Clips 42-1, 42-2, 42-3, 42-4, 42-5, 42-6, 42-7, 42-8**

PART IV   COMPLEX RECONSTRUCTIONS

43 Complex Reconstructions in Hand Surgery   249
Donald H. Lalonde, Jason Wong, Alistair Phillips, Nik Jagodzinski

▶ **Video Clips 43-1, 43-2, 43-3, 43-4, 43-5, 43-6, 43-7, 43-8, 43-9, 43-10, 43-11**

Index   253

Video Contents

PART II GENERAL PRINCIPLES OF WIDE AWAKE
HAND SURGERY

2   What Is Wide Awake Hand Surgery?
Alistair Phillips, Nik Jagodzinski, Donald H. Lalonde

Clip 2-1 Introduction to wide awake hand surgery.
Clip 2-2 Washing a contaminated hand in a wide awake patient in the
emergency department.

3   Safe Epinephrine in the Finger Means No Tourniquet
Donald H. Lalonde

Clip 3-1 History of the rise and fall of the epinephrine danger myth.
Clip 3-2 How to reverse epinephrine vasoconstriction with phentolamine
injection in the finger.

4   Tumescent Local Anesthesia
Donald H. Lalonde, Alistair Phillips, Duncan McGrouther

Clip 4-1 Principles of tumescent local anesthesia.

5   How to Inject Local Anesthetic With Minimal Pain
Donald H. Lalonde, Nik Jagodzinski, Alistair Phillips

Clip 5-1 How to inject local anesthetic with minimal pain.
Clip 5-2 Patient's pain impressions after a "hole-in-one" local anesthetic
injection for carpal tunnel surgery.
Clip 5-3 How and why to buffer lidocaine with epinephrine.
Clip 5-4 Cannula injection of tumescent local anesthetic for synovectomy
and tendon transfer.
Clip 5-5 How to perform a SIMPLE block.
Clip 5-6 A two dorsal injection block hurts more than a SIMPLE block.

6   Dealing With Systemic Adverse Reactions to Lidocaine
and Epinephrine
Donald H. Lalonde

Clip 6-1 Lowered epinephrine concentration for cardiac issues.
Clip 6-2 Managing the vasovagal fainting attack.

7 Tips on Talking to Your Patients About WALANT
Nik Jagodzinski, Alistair Phillips, Donald H. Lalonde

Clip 7-1 Explaining WALANT to a patient.
Clip 7-2 When patients are unsure about remaining awake.
Clip 7-3 Patient impression of pain of a local anesthetic needle versus an intravenous needle.

8 Talking With Patients During Surgery Saves Time
Donald H. Lalonde, Duncan McGrouther

Clip 8-1 Advice to patient during skin cancer excision in the hand.
Clip 8-2 During surgery the patient can verify that the deformity has been corrected.
Clip 8-3 Advice to a patient while K-wiring a finger fracture.
Clip 8-4 Advice to a 10-year-old during flexor tendon repair.
Clip 8-5 Giving intraoperative advice during carpal tunnel release.

9 WALANT Hand Surgery in Infants and Children
Donald H. Lalonde

Clip 9-1 Flexor tendon repair in a 6-year-old girl.
Clip 9-2 Flexor tendon repair in a 10-year-old girl.
Clip 9-3 Excision of a fifth finger nubbin in a 4-week-old infant.
Clip 9-4 Numbing a proximal phalanx fracture in a boy.

10 Field Sterility for Simple Cases Makes Sense
Donald H. Lalonde

Clip 10-1 Safety and value of field sterility for hand surgery.

12 The "Buy-In": Administration, Anesthesiology, Nursing, and Payers
Julie E. Adams, Michael W. Neumeister, Robert E. Van Demark, Jr., Carolyn L. Kerrigan, Peter C. Amadio, Donald H. Lalonde

Clip 12-1 Why patients love WALANT.

14 Scheduling Fifteen or More Hand Surgery Cases per Day
Donald H. Lalonde

Clip 14-1 Three carpal tunnel procedures performed per hour.

15 Integrating Hand Therapists Into WALANT
Susan Kean, Amanda Higgins, Donald H. Lalonde

Clip 15-1 Hand therapists in preoperative therapy consultation.
Clip 15-2 Patient watching structures being repaired.

Clip 15-3 Intraoperatively the surgeon and therapist teach the patient about postoperative care.

Clip 15-4 Therapist teaching a patient during flexor tendon repair surgery.

Clip 15-5 Allowing wrist extension and active flexion after flexor tendon repair.

Clip 15-6 Relative motion extension splinting for extensor tendon repair.

Clip 15-7 Early protected active motion after K-wired repair of finger fractures decided with the therapist during surgery.

Clip 15-8 Therapist teaching early movement 3 days after K-wiring finger fractures.

16 Minor Procedure Room Setup
Donald H. Lalonde, Geoff Cook

Clip 16-1 Clinic consultation and minor procedure room setup at the Saint John Regional Hospital.

Clip 16-2 Clinic consultation and minor procedure room setup at St. Joseph's Hospital.

Clip 16-3 Minor procedure accredited operating room at Dr. Lalonde's office.

PART III SPECIFIC DETAILS OF HOW TO PERFORM WIDE AWAKE HAND SURGERY FOR COMMON OPERATIONS

SECTION A AMPUTATION

17 Finger and Ray Amputation
Donald H. Lalonde

Clip 17-1 Local injection for proximal phalanx finger amputation.

Clip 17-2 SIMPLE block for distal phalanx squamous cell cancer amputation.

SECTION B NERVE DECOMPRESSION

18 Carpal Tunnel Decompression of the Median Nerve
Carolyn L. Kerrigan, Donald H. Lalonde, Shu Guo Xing, Jin Bo Tang

Clip 18-1 Patient impression of tourniquet with sedation versus WALANT for endoscopic carpal tunnel surgery.

Clip 18-2 A "hole-in-one" minimal pain local anesthetic injection for open carpal tunnel release.

Clip 18-3 Blunt-tipped cannula injection of local anesthetic for carpal tunnel surgery.

Clip 18-4 Injecting local anesthetic for endoscopic carpal tunnel release.

Clip 18-5 Patient consultation for carpal tunnel surgery.

Clip 18-6 Advising the patient after injection of local anesthetic for carpal tunnel release.

Clip 18-7 Intraoperative advice to the patient during carpal tunnel surgery.

Clip 18-8 Field sterility setup for open carpal tunnel release.

Clip 18-9 Carpal tunnel surgery (Lalonde).

Clip 18-10 Endoscopic carpal tunnel surgery.

19   Cubital Tunnel Decompression of the Ulnar Nerve
Donald H. Lalonde, Alistair Phillips

Clip 19-1 Checking for ulnar nerve subluxation with active movement during surgery.

Clip 19-2 How to inject local anesthetic for cubital tunnel release at the elbow.

Clip 19-3 Real-time injection of local anesthetic for cubital tunnel release.

Clip 19-4 Injecting for both cubital tunnel and carpal tunnel release in the same operation.

Clip 19-5 57 mm blunt-tipped 22-gauge cannula injection of local anesthetic for cubital tunnel release.

Clip 19-6 Prepping and draping for a WALANT cubital tunnel ulnar nerve release.

Clip 19-7 Cubital tunnel surgery with WALANT.

20   Lacertus Syndrome: Median Nerve Release at the Elbow
Elisabet Hagert, Donald H. Lalonde

Clip 20-1 What is lacertus syndrome?

Clip 20-2 Clinical examination of lacertus syndrome.

Clip 20-3 Local anesthetic injection for lacertus and carpal tunnel release.

Clip 20-4 Surgical release of lacertus fibrosus by Dr. Elisabet Hagert.

Clip 20-5 Lacertus and carpal tunnel injection and surgery by Dr. Don Lalonde.

SECTION C   TENDON DECOMPRESSION

21   Trigger Finger
Donald H. Lalonde

Clip 21-1 Trigger finger and thumb injection and surgery overview.

Clip 21-2 Injection of local anesthetic for trigger thumb surgery.

Clip 21-3 Trigger thumb surgery.

Clip 21-4 Wide awake trigger finger surgery

22   De Quervain Release
Donald H. Lalonde, Alistair Phillips

Clip 22-1 Injection and surgery for De Quervain synovitis. (Note that lignocaine is the same as lidocaine.)

SECTION D DUPUYTREN'S CONTRACTURE AND SOFT TISSUE EXCISION

23 Dupuytren's Contracture
Duncan McGrouther, Jason Wong, Donald H. Lalonde

Clip 23-1 Verifying active extension with active movement after cord resection.
Clip 23-2 Injecting local anesthetic for Dupuytren's surgery.

25 Small Soft Tissue Operations
Donald H. Lalonde, Jason Wong, Shu Guo Xing, Jin Bo Tang

Clip 25-1 Surgical sequence and result in an 89-year-old patient.
Clip 25-2 Excision lipoma on the forearm.

SECTION E ARTHRITIS SURGERY

26 Arthroplasty of the Proximal Interphalangeal Joint
Donald H. Lalonde

Clip 26-1 PIP arthroplasty.

27 Trapeziectomy With or Without Ligament Reconstruction for Thumb Basal Joint Arthritis
Donald H. Lalonde, Peter C. Amadio, Geoff Cook

Clip 27-1 Intraoperative decision-making about the appropriate procedure.
Clip 27-2 A patient with medical comorbidities compares local and general anesthesia.
Clip 27-3 Mixing the local anesthetic solution for a trapeziectomy.
Clip 27-4 Real-time 8-minute injection of a patient.
Clip 27-5 Cannula injection of local anesthetic for a trapeziectomy.
Clip 27-6 Ligament reconstruction with APL.
Clip 27-7 Watching the metacarpal move without grinding on scaphoid.
Clip 27-8 Patient impressions during trapeziectomy.

28 Thumb Metacarpophalangeal Joint Fusion and Ulnar Collateral Ligament Repair
Donald H. Lalonde

Clip 28-1 Local anesthetic injection for thumb MP fusion or UCL repair.
Clip 28-2 Thumb MP fusion in the same patient in Clip 28-1.
Clip 28-3 Thumb UCL repair.

Section F   Wrist Surgery

30   Wrist Arthroscopy
Elisabet Hagert, Donald H. Lalonde

Clip 30-1 Wrist arthroscopy.

31   Open Triangular Fibrocartilage Complex Repair
Elisabet Hagert, Donald H. Lalonde

Clip 31-1 Wide awake TFCC.

Section G   Lacerated Tendons and Tenolysis

32   Flexor Tendon Repair of the Finger
Jin Bo Tang, Shu Guo Xing, Jason Wong, Jeffrey Yao, Donald H. Lalonde

Clip 32-1 How WALANT has improved flexor tendon repair results.
Clip 32-2 Decreasing the rupture rate with intraoperative testing.
Clip 32-3 Tenolysis rate decreased by ensuring the repair fits through all pulleys.
Clip 32-4 Half a fist of true active movement.
Clip 32-5 Intraoperative patient education decreases rupture and tenolysis rates.
Clip 32-6 Determining whether to repair the superficialis.
Clip 32-7 How to inject local anesthetic for flexor tendon repair.
Clip 32-8 Dr. Jeffrey Yao has the patient see the fingers flex and extend.
Clip 32-9 Retrieving the tendon from the proximal flexor sheath.
Clip 32-10 Delivering a misdirected FDP proximal stump between both slips of FDS.
Clip 32-11 Suturing tendon inside flexor tendon sheath.
Clip 32-12 Total A4 pulley venting with no bowstringing.
Clip 32-13 Testing flexor pollicis longus repair during surgery.
Clip 32-14 Where and how to dissect in pulp of distal phalanx to avoid numbness.
Clip 32-15 Passive and active finger movement up to half a fist after surgery.
Clip 32-16 Profundus glides 1 cm of tendon when patient makes half a fist.
Clip 32-17 Tendon repair caught on proximal edge of A4 pulley.
Clip 32-18 Fiona Peck Manchester short splint and Gwen van Strien scratch movement for true active movement after flexor tendon repair.

34   Flexor Tendon Repair of the Forearm
Donald H. Lalonde

Clip 34-1 "Spaghetti wrist." Active movement in proximal forearm identifies which proximal tendons belong to which distal tendon ends.

35 Extensor Tendon Repair of the Finger
Donald H. Lalonde

Clip 35-1 Relative motion extension splint decreases excursion in extensor tendon repair in the proximal finger.

Clip 35-2 Merritt relative motion flexion splinting for boutonniere deformity.

Clip 35-3 WALANT mallet fracture management.

Clip 35-4 Percutaneous extensor tendon repair.

Clip 35-5 Pencil test for relative motion splinting.

36 Extensor Tendon Repair of the Hand
Donald H. Lalonde, Geoff Cook

Clip 36-1 Hand extensor repair revolutionized by Merritt relative motion extension splinting.

Clip 36-2 Extensors reflexively relax when patient is asked to actively flex the finger.

37 Extensor Tendon Repair of the Forearm
Donald H. Lalonde

Clip 37-1 Three different extensor tendon repairs of the forearm.

38 Tenolysis
Jason Wong, Michael Sauerbier, Peter C. Amadio, Donald H. Lalonde

Clip 38-1 Dr. Jason Wong performs tenolysis after finger amputation.

Clip 38-2 Dr. Michael Sauerbier performs tenolysis.

Clip 38-3 Tenolysis after finger fracture.

Clip 38-4 Tenolysis in a 63-year-old woman who had been unable to flex her long and ring fingers since a tendon repair at age 3.

Clip 38-5 Patient ruptures her own adhesions in the extensor tendons after wrist fusion.

SECTION H TENDON TRANSFERS

39 Tendon Transfers
Donald H. Lalonde, Robert M. Szabo, Mark E. Baratz

Clip 39-1 EI to EPL: getting the transfer tension right; clinical experience.

Clip 39-2 Dr. Robert Szabo performs a wide awake EI to EPL transfer.

Clip 39-3 Dr. Mark Baratz demonstrates a patient watching herself extend her thumb.

Clip 39-4 How to inject local anesthetic for EI to EPL transfer.

Clip 39-5 EI to EPL surgery with intraoperative testing of thumb flexion and extension.

Clip 39-6 Another video of EI to EPL surgery with intraoperative testing of thumb flexion and extension.

Clip 39-7 FDS4 to FPL transfer with radius plate removal.

Clip 39-8 84-year-old man with cardiac issues was given a lowered epinephrine concentration.

SECTION I   LACERATED NERVES

40   Lacerated Nerves
Donald H. Lalonde

Clip 40-1 Relative motion flexion splint.

SECTION J   FRACTURES

41   Finger Fractures
Donald H. Lalonde

Clip 41-1 Early protected movement 3 days after K-wiring middle phalanx fracture.

Clip 41-2 Two finger fractures: numbing, intraoperative testing of functionally stable fixation of K-wire reduction, early protected movement demonstration, and final result.

Clip 41-3 Augmented field sterility setup for inserting K-wires in a minor procedure room.

Clip 41-4 Real-time minimal pain local injection for proximal phalanx fracture.

Clip 41-5 Advice to an awake patient at the end of finger fracture reduction surgery.

Clip 41-6 Testing stability of dorsal blocking K-wire for dorsal fracture dislocation of PIP joint.

Clip 41-7 Wide awake operative reduction of a 4-week-old scissoring malunion of the proximal phalanx.

Clip 41-8 Distraction splint for comminuted PIP and MP fractures.

Clip 41-9 Fracture boutonniere treated with a relative motion flexion splint only.

Clip 41-10 Mallet fractures involving 50% to 60% of the joint but with congruous or parallel joint surfaces (not subluxated) can be treated with mallet splinting only.

42   Reduction and Internal Fixation of Metacarpal Fractures
Shu Guo Xing, Jin Bo Tang, Donald H. Lalonde

Clip 42-1 Fracture dislocation at the base of the thumb metacarpal (Bennett fracture).

Clip 42-2 Fracture dislocation at the base of the fifth metacarpal.

Clip 42-3 Local anesthesia for fourth and fifth metacarpal operative reduction.

Clip 42-4 Local anesthetic injection for WALANT metacarpal plate removal.

Clip 42-5 Operative reduction of fourth and fifth metacarpal fractures in the patient injected with local anesthetic seen in Clip 42-3.

Clip 42-6 Early protected movement 3 days after K-wire fixation of a metacarpal fracture.

Clip 42-7 A 3-month-old malunion of a metacarpal with intraoperative testing of full flexion and extension after reduction and plating.

Clip 42-8 Checking scissoring after dynamic compression bone clamp metacarpal fracture reduction.

PART IV   COMPLEX RECONSTRUCTIONS

43   Complex Reconstructions in Hand Surgery
Donald H. Lalonde, Jason Wong, Alistair Phillips, Nik Jagodzinski

Clip 43-1 Repair of a 5½-week-old FPL laceration.

Clip 43-2 Change thumb tip pinch after adult pollicization.

Clip 43-3 Cleaning a severely contaminated hand wound in the emergency
department.

Clip 43-4 Extensor tendon graft of the dorsum of the hand.

Clip 43-5 FCR and FCU transfer in a polio case.

Clip 43-6 Finger revascularization with wrist vein grafts by Dr. Jason Wong.

Clip 43-7 Homodigital island flap by Dr. Jason Wong.

Clip 43-8 Restoration of thumb extension after subtotal amputation.

Clip 43-9 Ruptured FPL repair under the motor branch in the carpal tunnel.

Clip 43-10 Swan neck FDS transfer.

Clip 43-11 Palmaris longus tendon graft for rupture of fourth and fifth
extensors.

Part I

Atlas of Tumescent Local Anesthesia With Forearm, Wrist, Hand, and Finger Injections

CHAPTER 1

ATLAS OF IMAGES OF LOCAL ANESTHETIC DIFFUSION ANATOMY

Donald H. Lalonde

In this atlas, the images you will see are drawn from photographs of live human volunteers injected with tumescent local anesthesia to determine where the solution naturally diffuses when you inject it under the skin in the hand, wrist, and forearm.

Producing tumescing local anesthesia requires injecting enough volume of anesthetic solution—lidocaine (also called lignocaine) with epinephrine— under the skin so that you can see its swelling, and you can feel it when you palpate the area (see Chapter 4). It is a form of extravascular Bier block injected only where you intend to operate.

In addition to anatomic maps of where the local anesthetic diffuses when you inject it in one place in the forearm, wrist, and hand, this chapter also describes the natural barriers to local anesthetic diffusion formed by creases and glabrous/nonglabrous skin boundaries.

GUIDE TO THE ATLAS

- Each image answers the following question: Where does the local anesthetic diffuse and have its numbing effect when you inject it under the skin without moving the needle in the *red injection point* of the illustrated area?

- The *blue areas* show the diffusion of visible and palpable lidocaine with epinephrine that usually takes place within 30 minutes after injection in most patients. These blue areas will be both numbed and vasoconstricted.

- The *green areas* are blocked by nerve block. They may take up to an hour or longer after injection to achieve the peak nerve block. These green areas will not be vasoconstricted. Bleeding in the green areas may be more than in normal skin because of the sympathectomy effect of the nerve blocks. To avoid bleeding in the green areas, simply inject more local anesthetic where you will dissect, as described in Chapter 4.

- Note that the ligaments at the glabrous/nonglabrous skin junction act as a diffusion barrier to distribution of the local anesthetic. This is where the volar skin meets the dorsal skin of the hand. This also is the embryologic boundary/border of many nerve distributions.

- Ligaments that create creases in the hand and fingers also act as a natural diffusion barrier to local anesthetic. You will usually have to inject on both sides of the creases.

3

- Preexisting scars and lacerations create natural diffusion barriers to local anesthetic. You will usually have to inject on both sides of preexisting scars and lacerations.
- As in all anatomy, different patients will have small differences. Not all patients will get the green distal nerve blocks.

MIDLINE DORSAL FOREARM

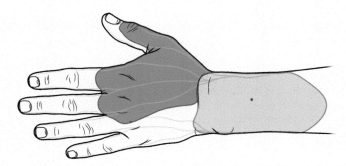

When you inject 20 ml of 1% lidocaine with 1:100,000 epinephrine (buffered at a ratio of 10 ml of lidocaine/epinephrine to 1 ml of 8.4% sodium bicarbonate) 10 cm proximal to the wrist crease in the dorsal forearm midline in the red injection point just under the skin without moving the needle, local anesthetic can be seen and palpated to diffuse in the blue area in an unscarred patient. You numb the green area by nerve block, but this area has no epinephrine vasoconstriction and may bleed more because of the sympathectomy of the nerve block.

MIDLINE VOLAR FOREARM

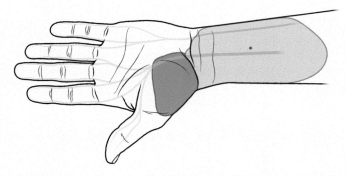

When you inject 20 ml of 1% lidocaine with 1:100,000 epinephrine (buffered at a ratio of 10 ml of lidocaine/epinephrine to 1 ml of 8.4% sodium bicarbonate) 10 cm proximal to the wrist crease in the volar forearm midline in the red injection point just under the skin without moving the needle, local anesthetic can be seen and palpated to diffuse in the blue area in an unscarred patient. You numb the green area by nerve block, but this area has no epinephrine vasoconstriction and may bleed more because of the sympathectomy of the nerve block. The median and ulnar nerves may not be blocked unless the needle gets beneath the deep forearm fascia, since this can act as a natural barrier to local anesthetic diffusion.

MIDLINE RADIAL FOREARM

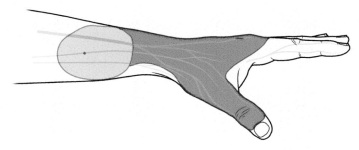

When you inject 20 ml of 1% lidocaine with 1:100,000 epinephrine (buffered at a ratio of 10 ml of lidocaine/epinephrine to 1 ml of 8.4% sodium bicarbonate) 10 cm proximal to the wrist crease in the radial forearm midline in the red injection point just under the skin without moving the needle, local anesthetic can be seen and palpated to diffuse in the blue area in an unscarred patient. You numb the green area by nerve block, but this area has no epinephrine vasoconstriction and may bleed more because of the sympathectomy of the nerve block.

MIDLINE ULNAR FOREARM

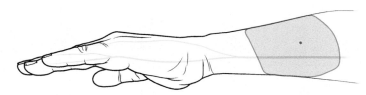

When you inject 20 ml of 1% lidocaine with 1:100,000 epinephrine (buffered at a ratio of 10 ml of lidocaine/epinephrine to 1 ml of 8.4% sodium bicarbonate) 10 cm proximal to the wrist crease in the ulnar forearm midline in the red injection point just under the skin without moving the needle, local anesthetic can be seen and palpated to diffuse in the blue area in an unscarred patient.

MIDLINE VOLAR WRIST

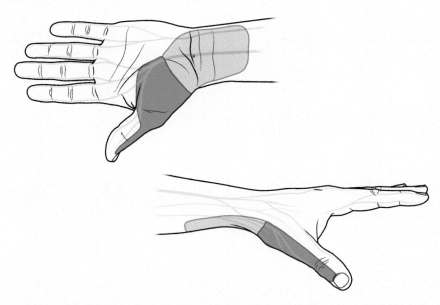

When you inject 10 ml of 1% lidocaine with 1:100,000 epinephrine (buffered at a ratio of 10 ml of lidocaine/epinephrine to 1 ml of 8.4% sodium bicarbonate) in the midvolar wrist in the red injection point just under the skin without moving the needle, local anesthetic can be seen and palpated to diffuse in the blue area in an unscarred patient. When the injection is under the skin and not below the forearm fascia, you may not achieve a median or ulnar nerve block, since the deep forearm fascia can act as a natural diffusion barrier to local anesthetic diffusion. You do get a palmar cutaneous and a dorsal sensory block, as shown in green. More of the local anesthetic tracks proximally, because the wrist crease acts as a natural barrier to local anesthetic diffusion into the palm. You numb the green area by nerve block, but this area has no epinephrine vasoconstriction and may bleed more because of the sympathectomy of the nerve block.

MIDLINE DORSAL WRIST

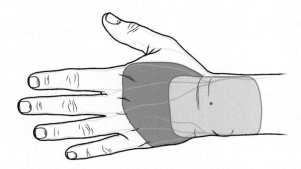

When you inject 10 ml of 1% lidocaine with 1:100,000 epinephrine (buffered at a ratio of 10 ml of lidocaine/epinephrine to 1 ml of 8.4% sodium bicarbonate) in the middorsal wrist in the red injection point just under the skin without moving the needle, local anesthetic can be seen and palpated to diffuse in the blue area in an unscarred patient. You numb the green area by nerve block, but this area has no epinephrine vasoconstriction and may bleed more because of the sympathectomy of the nerve block.

MIDLINE RADIAL WRIST

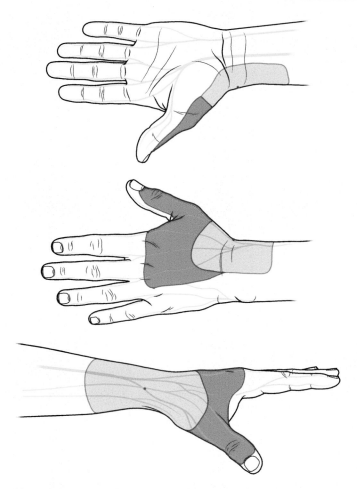

When you inject 10 ml of 1% lidocaine with 1:100,000 epinephrine (buffered at a ratio of 10 ml of lidocaine/epinephrine to 1 ml of 8.4% sodium bicarbonate) in the midradial wrist in the red injection point just under the skin without moving the needle, local anesthetic can be seen and palpated to diffuse in the blue area in an unscarred patient. You numb the green area by nerve block, but this area has no epinephrine vasoconstriction and may bleed more because of the sympathectomy of the nerve block.

MIDLINE ULNAR WRIST

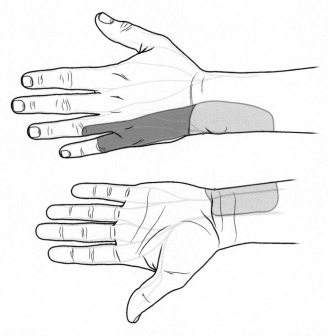

When you inject 10 ml of 1% lidocaine with 1:100,000 epinephrine (buffered at a ratio of 10 ml of lidocaine/epinephrine to 1 ml of 8.4% sodium bicarbonate) in the midulnar wrist in the red injection point just under the skin without moving the needle, local anesthetic can be seen and palpated to diffuse in the blue area in an unscarred patient. You numb the green area by nerve block, but this area has no epinephrine vasoconstriction and may bleed more because of the sympathectomy of the nerve block.

MIDPALMAR HAND

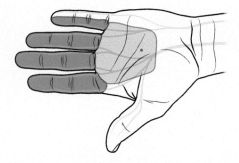

When you inject 10 ml of 1% lidocaine with 1:100,000 epinephrine (buffered at a ratio of 10 ml of lidocaine/epinephrine to 1 ml of 8.4% sodium bicarbonate) in the midpalm in the red injection point just under the skin without moving the needle, local anesthetic can be seen and palpated to diffuse in the blue area in an unscarred patient. The green areas are numbed by nerve block, but these areas have no epinephrine vasoconstriction and may bleed more because of the sympathectomy of the nerve block.

MIDDORSAL HAND

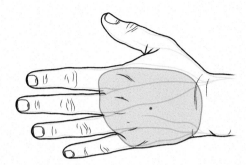

When you inject 10 ml of 1% lidocaine with 1:100,000 epinephrine (buffered at a ratio of 10 ml of lidocaine/epinephrine to 1 ml of 8.4% sodium bicarbonate) in the dorsum of the midhand in the red injection point just under the skin without moving the needle, local anesthetic can be seen and palpated to diffuse in the blue area in an unscarred patient. The proximal phalanx dorsal skin may not be blocked past the web space.

ULNAR HAND

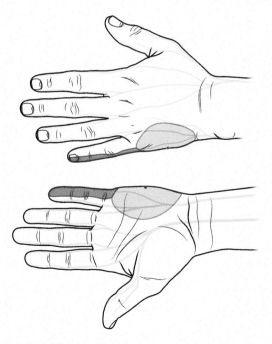

When you inject 10 ml of 1% lidocaine with 1:100,000 epinephrine (buffered at a ratio of 10 ml of lidocaine/epinephrine to 1 ml of 8.4% sodium bicarbonate) in the ulnar midhand in the red injection point just under the skin without moving the needle, local anesthetic can be seen and palpated to diffuse in the blue area in an unscarred patient. You numb the green area by nerve block, but this area has no epinephrine vasoconstriction and may bleed more because of the sympathectomy of the nerve block.

THUMB MIDMETACARPAL DORSAL

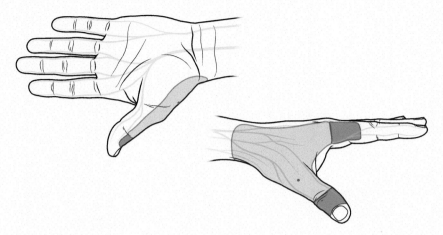

When you inject 10 ml of 1% lidocaine with 1:100,000 epinephrine (buffered at a ratio of 10 ml of lidocaine/epinephrine to 1 ml of 8.4% sodium bicarbonate) in the dorsum of the midmetacarpal thumb in the red injection point just under the skin without moving the needle, local anesthetic can be seen and palpated to diffuse in the blue area in an unscarred patient. Note that the ligaments at the glabrous/nonglabrous skin junction act as a natural diffusion barrier to volar distribution of the local anesthetic. The interphalangeal thumb crease also acts as a natural barrier to local anesthetic diffusion. The green areas are numbed by nerve block, but these areas have no epinephrine vaso-constriction and may bleed more because of the sympathectomy of the nerve block.

THUMB MIDMETACARPAL VOLAR

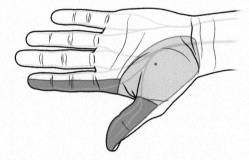

When you inject 10 ml of 1% lidocaine with 1:100,000 epinephrine (buffered at a ratio of 10 ml of lidocaine/epinephrine to 1 ml of 8.4% sodium bicarbonate) in the volar aspect of the midmetacar-pal thumb red injection point just under the skin without moving the needle, local anesthetic can be seen and palpated to diffuse in the blue area in an unscarred patient. Note that the ligaments at the glabrous/nonglabrous skin junction act as a diffusion barrier to dorsal distribution of the local an-esthetic. The thenar eminence creases in the palm also act as a barrier to local anesthetic diffusion. The green areas are numbed by nerve block, but these areas have no epinephrine vasoconstriction and may bleed more because of the sympathectomy of the nerve block.

SINGLE SUBCUTANEOUS INJECTION IN THE MIDLINE PROXIMAL PHALANX WITH LIDOCAINE AND EPINEPHRINE (SIMPLE) FINGER BLOCK

- SIMPLE is the acronym for *single subcutaneous injection in the midline proximal phalanx with lidocaine and epinephrine.*

- See the clip of SIMPLE block injection in Chapter 17.

- Only 2 ml is required for a good digital block.

- There is level II evidence that patients prefer this block to the two dorsal injection block.[1]

- There is level I evidence that needle penetration of the palmar skin is not more painful than needle penetration of web space skin.[2]

- There is level II evidence that this block hurts less if you inject it over 60 seconds than if you inject it over 10 seconds.[3]

- There is level II evidence that lidocaine without epinephrine digital blocks last 5 hours, whereas lidocaine with epinephrine blocks last 10 hours.[4]

- There is level I evidence that the pain-relieving effect of bupivacaine blocks lasts 15 hours, whereas the annoying numbness to touch and pressure lasts more than 30 hours with these blocks.[5]

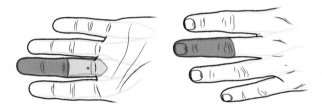

When you inject 2 ml of 1% lidocaine with 1:100,000 epinephrine (buffered at a ratio of 10 ml of lidocaine/epinephrine to 1 ml of 8.4% sodium bicarbonate) in subcutaneous fat in the red injection point just under the skin without moving the needle, local anesthetic can be seen and palpated to diffuse in the blue area in an unscarred patient. The two digital nerves always get numb. You numb the green area by nerve block, but this area has no epinephrine vasoconstriction and may bleed more because of the sympathectomy of the nerve block.

"SIMPLE" FINGER BLOCK WITH DORSAL BLOCK AUGMENTATION

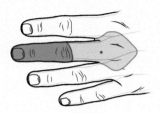

When you inject 2 ml of 1% lidocaine with 1:100,000 epinephrine (buffered at a ratio of 10 ml of lidocaine/epinephrine to 1 ml of 8.4% sodium bicarbonate) in subcutaneous fat in the red injection point just under the skin without moving the needle, local anesthetic can be seen and palpated to diffuse in the blue area in an unscarred patient. The green areas are numbed by nerve block, but these areas have no epinephrine vasoconstriction and may bleed more because of the sympathectomy of the nerve block.

"SIMPLE" THUMB BLOCK

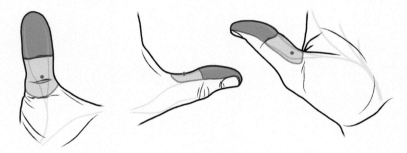

When you inject 2 ml of 1% lidocaine with 1:100,000 epinephrine (buffered at a ratio of 10 ml of lidocaine/epinephrine to 1 ml of 8.4% sodium bicarbonate) in subcutaneous fat in the red injection point just under the skin without moving the needle, local anesthetic can be seen and palpated to diffuse in the blue area in an unscarred patient. The two digital nerves always get numb. You numb the green area by nerve block, but this area has no epinephrine vasoconstriction and may bleed more because of the sympathectomy of the nerve block.

DORSAL THUMB PROXIMAL PHALANX BLOCK

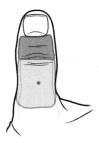

When you inject 2 ml of 1% lidocaine with 1:100,000 epinephrine (buffered at a ratio of 10 ml of lidocaine/epinephrine to 1 ml of 8.4% sodium bicarbonate) in subcutaneous fat in the red injection point just under the skin without moving the needle, local anesthetic can be seen and palpated to diffuse in the blue area in an unscarred patient. You numb the green area by nerve block, but this area has no epinephrine vasoconstriction and may bleed more because of the sympathectomy of the nerve block.

References

1. Williams JG, Lalonde DH. Randomized comparison of the single-injection volar subcutaneous block and the two-injection dorsal block for digital anesthesia. Plast Reconstr Surg 118:1195, 2006.
2. Wheelock ME, Leblanc M, Chung B, Williams J, Lalonde DH. Is it true that injecting palmar finger skin hurts more than dorsal skin? New level I evidence. Hand (N Y) 6:47, 2011.
3. Hamelin ND, St-Amand H, Lalonde DH, Harris PG, Brutus JP. Decreasing the pain of finger block injection: level II evidence. Hand (N Y) 8:69, 2013.
4. Thomson CJ, Lalonde DH. Randomized double-blind comparison of duration of anesthesia among three commonly used agents in digital nerve block. Plast Reconstr Surg 118:429, 2006.
5. Calder K, Chung B, O'Brien C, Lalonde DH. Bupivacaine digital blocks: How long is the pain relief and temperature elevation? Plast Reconstr Surg 131:1098, 2013.

Part II

GENERAL PRINCIPLES OF WIDE AWAKE
HAND SURGERY

CHAPTER 2

WHAT IS WIDE AWAKE HAND SURGERY?

Alistair Phillips, Nik Jagodzinski, Donald H. Lalonde

Wide awake hand surgery is well described by its other name, *WALANT,* which stands for *w*ide *a*wake *l*ocal *a*nesthesia *no t*ourniquet. The only two medications most patients are given for wide awake hand surgery are lidocaine for anesthesia and epinephrine for hemostasis. We inject tumescent lidocaine and epinephrine in large enough volumes to be visible or palpable wherever dissection will be done (see Chapter 3). This is a form of extravascular Bier block injected only where you need it, but without the painful tourniquet.

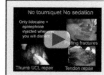

Clip 2-1 Introduction to wide awake hand surgery.

- Lidocaine and epinephrine are probably two of the safest and most widely tested injectable drugs that are used in humans (see Chapters 3 and 6). Dentists have injected billions of doses of these two medications in their offices since 1950 with no preoperative testing, no monitoring, no intravenous insertion, and very few adverse events.

- Like dental procedures, we can perform wide awake hand surgery with no preoperative testing, no insertion of an intravenous line, and no monitoring, because the only medications we inject are lidocaine and epinephrine. After the procedure, the patient simply gets up and goes home.

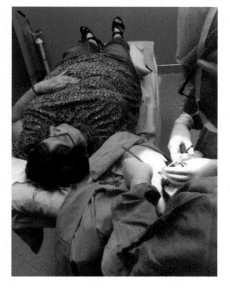

Cubital tunnel release with WALANT.

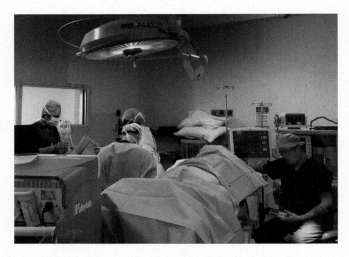

Traditional surgery performed with general anesthesia and a tourniquet.

PATIENTS LOVE WALANT

- They have no nausea, vomiting, urinary retention, or other unwanted side effects associated with opiates or sedation.

- They spend less time at the hospital for the procedure, because postoperative recovery time is just minutes, since they receive no sedation and no opioid medications. They can just get up and go home, as they would do after a visit to the dentist.

- They have no need to have someone stay with them the evening after the surgery. Following outpatient procedures with general anesthesia in many facilities, patients are required to have a responsible adult stay with them for 12 to 24 hours. This is difficult for many patients, especially if they have children.

- Patients get to know and talk to their surgeon during the surgery for advice on how to care for the hand postoperatively, time off work, and other issues.

- There is no downtime from work or need for a babysitter when they go for preoperative testing for sedation on a day before the surgery.

- Hand surgery under pure local anesthesia is not expensive. Many patients in developing countries could afford hand surgery if they did not have to pay the large costs associated with sedation and general anesthesia in the main operating room.

- Patients do not have to obtain an unnecessary ECG or chest radiographs, attend an anesthesia consultation, or undergo preoperative blood tests.

- There is no unnecessary insertion with a 20-gauge intravenous cannula. All the patient will feel is a single brief prick with a 27- or 30-gauge needle in the hand when the local anesthetic is injected (see Chapter 5).

- Patients can see repaired structures working during the surgery after a loss of function such as tendon laceration, tenolysis, tendon transfer, hand fracture, or Dupuytren's contracture. This visual memory helps motivate them throughout postoperative therapy and recovery.

- Patients do not need to endure a tourniquet for even 5 minutes. We tell all our trainees that they need to put a tourniquet on their own arm or forearm for 5 minutes before they ever say, "Patients tolerate it well." The true meaning of this phrase might be, "Patients let me do it, even though it hurts."

- The fact that there is no need for a tourniquet is advantageous in patients who have lymphedema or arteriovenous shunts in the forearm.

- Patients do not need to fast or change medication schedules before the procedure, which is particularly helpful for diabetic patients.

- Patients with sore elbows, shoulders, or backs can position themselves comfortably for hand and elbow surgery, because there is no tourniquet or anesthesiology equipment preventing them from shifting out of an uncomfortable position. They can easily turn on their side during the procedure.

- Patients do not need to get undressed for surgery when we use field sterility.

- WALANT is safer for patients than sedation, especially for individuals with medical comorbidities. All anesthesiologists agree that less sedation is safer sedation. The safest sedation is no sedation.

- Surgeons are less likely to operate on the wrong hand or the wrong finger if the patient is wide awake with no sedation.

- Trauma patients can undergo surgery during the day in minor procedure rooms instead of in the middle of the night in the main operating room. They do not need hospital admission to wait for or recover from sedation. Surgeons and nurses are more likely to be able to perform surgery well when rested during daytime hours than while tired at night.

- There is no need to discontinue anticoagulation medication in most cases, because the epinephrine provides enough hemostasis that the wound dries up nicely.

- It is possible to see a patient in consultation and operate on him or her the same day, because there is little to no preoperative workup required for pure local anesthesia. This is much less expensive and more convenient for patients who have to travel long distances to the surgeon's clinic or office.

SURGEONS LOVE WALANT

- We can make adjustments on repaired tendons and finger fractures after seeing active movement in comfortable, cooperative patients and make certain everything is working well before we close the skin. This decreases the rate of rupture and tenolysis after flexor tendon repair.

- Patients help to rupture adhesions in tenolysis and remember what they achieve in motion at surgery when they are unsedated.

- We have an easier time setting proper tension on tendon transfers before we close the skin by watching the patient move the transfer to test the tension.

- We see what is happening with active movement during the surgery in complex reconstructive cases to improve results.

- We do not have to look after patients who must be admitted to the hospital after hand surgery because of sedation complications such as nausea and vomiting.

- We can operate on patients with multiple medical problems safely and easily, because we give them no sedation. They walk in, have their hand surgery, and then get up and go home with their medical issues unchanged. The fact that they are morbidly obese, diabetic, or have severe lung disease has no bearing on the hand surgery itself, only on the sedation.

- We do not have to use cautery for most cases because epinephrine hemostasis is very good. We only open cautery as required, not as a routine. The epinephrine and natural clotting typically dries up the field by the time we get to skin closure. This can reduce operative time and the cost of cautery equipment, and possibly even prevent postoperative hematoma.

- There is no need to stop let-down bleeding from a tourniquet, because we do not use one.

- We do not need to stop anticoagulation therapy in many if not most cases, because epinephrine hemostasis is good. This is safer for the patient and decreases the liability for the surgeon.

- We have an easier time in patients with lymphedema, dialysis access, or previous vascular surgery in which a tourniquet might cause problems.

- We get to educate the patient during the surgery for better outcomes and fewer complications. Time spent on intraoperative patient education can decrease the time spent in the office on patient education (see Chapters 7 and 8). Patients tend to remember the intraoperative advice, which leads to fewer complications.

- Patient compliance is improved. When you personally tell patients to keep their hand elevated and immobile at the end of the surgery, they are more likely to comply than if a nurse tells them this in the recovery room when they are still under the influence of sedatives.

- We only need one nurse for most simple hand operations, such as carpal tunnel release. This greatly increases efficiency and productivity and reduces costs (see Chapter 14). We can perform more cases in the same amount of time at less cost. It is never necessary to wait for the slowest member of a big team to finish his or her work so we can proceed.

- Simple operations such as carpal tunnel and trigger finger can be moved out of the main operating room. We can perform them in the clinic or office with field sterility for greatly improved turnover time and patient convenience (see Chapter 10).

- We can perform hand trauma procedures such as tendon repair and finger fracture with K-wiring during the day in minor procedure rooms instead of in the middle of the night in the main operating room.

- We can use lidocaine with epinephrine injection to flood the area, even in sedated or sleeping patients, to decrease bleeding and pain at the end of surgery. Many of us use lidocaine and epinephrine without a tourniquet, even when we have patients under general anesthesia.

- We can wash very dirty hand injuries in the emergency department with tap water after numbing the hand. The concentration of bacteria in running tap water is negligibly higher than sterile saline solution in countries where water cleanliness is highly regulated.

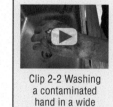

Clip 2-2 Washing a contaminated hand in a wide awake patient in the emergency department.

WHY NO SEDATION?

- There is no need for sedation for many if not most patients: the only two reasons patients needed sedation in the past for hand surgery were (1) to tolerate the pain of the tourniquet and (2) to tolerate the pain of injection of the local anesthetic. Those reasons are no longer valid, because the use of epinephrine has removed the need for a tourniquet (see Chapter 3), and local anesthetic can be reliably injected in an almost pain-free manner (see Chapter 5).

- Sedated patients cannot remember intraoperative teaching from their surgeon and will miss this excellent communication opportunity because of the amnestic drugs.

- Some patients become uninhibited and harder to manage with small amounts of sedation and end up requiring general anesthesia, with all its inconveniences.

- Pain-free, unsedated, cooperative patients can move their reconstructed fingers through a full range of motion during the surgery and remember how well the reconstructed hand functions. The surgeon can make changes during the procedure to improve the outcome, and patients are motivated to achieve the same movement they remember seeing on the operating table.

CONCLUSION

Wide awake hand surgery is being practiced by an increasing number of hand surgeons in most countries of the world. This will only increase in the future, because this technique is safer, more convenient for patients and surgeons, and much more affordable. Most surgeons who have tried it continue to use it.

CHAPTER 3

SAFE EPINEPHRINE IN THE FINGER MEANS NO TOURNIQUET

Donald H. Lalonde

THE RISE AND FALL OF THE MYTH OF THE DANGER OF INJECTING EPINEPHRINE IN THE FINGER

In the period before 1950, the belief developed among surgeons that epinephrine causes finger necrosis. This dogma became entrenched in medical school teachings, where we were told that we should not inject epinephrine into "fingers, nose, penis, and toes." Evidence-based medicine has now altered that misconception. This chapter tells the story of how it happened.

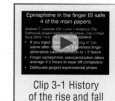

Clip 3-1 History of the rise and fall of the epinephrine danger myth.

THE LONG HISTORY OF SAFE USE OF EPINEPHRINE IN THE FINGER BY CANADIAN SURGEONS

- When I was a medical student at Queen's University in Kingston, Ontario, from 1975 to 1979, there was an excellent hand surgeon, Dr. Pat Shoemaker, who used epinephrine in the finger all of the time. He did wide awake flexor tendon repair with field sterility in the emergency department and got good results. Some of his colleagues were skeptical and taught medical students the traditional view that epinephrine in the finger was dangerous and could cause finger necrosis as a result of vasoconstriction. Only Dr. Shoemaker was "allowed" to do it, because he was a hand surgeon who did not have trouble—"yet!" He never did get into trouble, and has long since retired and passed away.

- Dr. Bob MacFarlane of London, Ontario, past president of the American Society for Surgery of the Hand, became famous for his Dupuytren's research. He regularly performed wide awake Dupuytren's surgery with lidocaine and epinephrine hemostasis.

- Dr. John Fielding, the first plastic surgeon in Ottawa, pioneered use of wide awake hand surgery with epinephrine hemostasis in that city. Many Ottawa surgeons followed his lead and used the technique routinely long before I did.

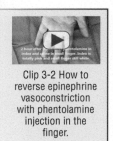

Clip 3-2 How to
reverse epinephrine
vasoconstriction
with phentolamine
injection in the
finger.

- Many other Canadian hand surgeons in other cities adopted the same technique.

SIX THINGS STIMULATED MY INTEREST IN BEGINNING ROUTINE ELECTIVE EPINEPHRINE HEMOSTASIS USE IN THE FINGER FOR EVERY CASE IN 2001

1. I knew of well over 100 surgeon-years of clinical safety in the practices of Drs. Shoemaker, MacFarlane, Fielding, and others who routinely injected epinephrine in fingers. These were good surgeons. I trusted and respected their clinical judgment.

2. I knew I could use phentolamine as an epinephrine vasoconstriction rescue agent if I needed it.

3. I had been using epinephrine for carpal tunnel, flexor sheath ganglion, and trigger finger procedures for many years with no problems.

4. I had used epinephrine in the finger many times before 2001, but not routinely, and I had not encountered any problems.

5. We had great difficulty getting the main operating room for our hand trauma cases because of a chronic shortage of anesthesiologists in Saint John. Epinephrine hemostasis meant no tourniquet was required. It also meant we could operate on a patient with a traumatic hand injury outside the main operating room at our convenience, Monday through Friday, 9 to 5, without having to admit patients or wait for an anesthesiologist.

6. Dr. Keith Denkler published his landmark paper in 2001.[1] Dr. Denkler painstakingly reviewed 120 years of literature from 1880 to 2000, most of it by hand through *Index Medicus* volumes, and *did not find one case* of lidocaine with epinephrine finger necrosis in the world literature. This was my tipping point. After reading his paper, I decided to use epinephrine in every finger with good capillary refill on fingertip pulp palpation until I needed phentolamine rescue.

FOUR MAIN CONCEPTS THAT SUPPORT THE FALL OF THE MYTH

1. We can reliably reverse epinephrine vasoconstriction with phentolamine in the human finger.[2]

2. There were no lost fingers and not one case required phentolamine rescue in a prospective study of 3110 consecutive cases of elective

epinephrine injection in the finger and hand by nine surgeons in six cities, called the *Dalhousie Project clinical phase*.[3] A similar study of over 1111 fingers injected with epinephrine in 2010 by another group of surgeons yielded similar results.[4]

3. More than 100 cases of high-dose 1:1000 epinephrine[5,6] revealed that not one finger injected with a dosage 100 times the concentration of epinephrine that we use clinically actually died. If 1:1000 epinephrine does not kill fingers, it is highly unlikely that 1:100,000 will ever kill a finger.

4. The source of the epinephrine myth, created between 1920 and 1945, stemmed from the use of procaine (Novocaine).[7] It was the "new caine," invented in 1903 to add to existing cocaine. It was the only safely injectable local anesthetic until the introduction of lidocaine in 1948. More fingers died from procaine injection alone than from procaine plus epinephrine injection. Procaine started with a pH of 3.6 and became more acidic as it sat on the shelf.[8,9] The U.S. Food and Drug Administration (FDA) instituted mandatory expiration dates on injectable medicines in 1979.[10] The "smoking gun" paper that established that procaine was the actual cause of finger deaths that had been blamed on epinephrine was a 1948 FDA warning published in the *Journal of the American Medical Association* that found batches of procaine with a pH of 1 destined for injection into humans![11]

HOW TO REVERSE EPINEPHRINE VASOCONSTRICTION IN THE HUMAN FINGER WITH PHENTOLAMINE

• I have now injected more than 2000 fingers with epinephrine. I have not needed phentolamine rescue once. I also have been treating patients with morphine for over 30 years and have not had to rescue one with naloxone. That does not mean I will not in the future, and I know how to use it if I need it.

• I have demonstrated phentolamine rescue to many visiting surgeons. I recommend that all hand surgeons try it at least once. This will help them and their nursing colleagues dissolve their epinephrine fear.

• What is phentolamine? Phentolamine is an alpha-adrenergic blocking agent introduced in 1957 as an antihypertensive agent in pheochromocytoma management.

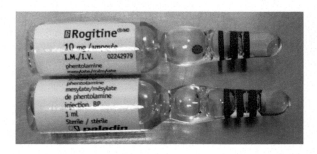

Phentolamine (Rogitine) is the rescue agent for epinephrine vasoconstriction in the human finger.

- Phentolamine manufacturers recommend a dosage of phentolamine of 5 mg intravenously to lower blood pressure.[12] The dosage to reverse adrenaline vasoconstriction in the finger is to inject 1 mg of phentolamine in 1 ml or more of saline solution into the subcutaneous fat wherever there is severe epinephrine pallor in the skin. This small extravascular dose will not affect blood pressure. The finger will pink up within an hour or two.

THE DALHOUSIE PROJECT EXPERIMENTAL PHASE

We needed to prove that phentolamine did in fact reliably reverse epinephrine vasoconstriction in the human finger. In Halifax in 2002, we performed a prospective, randomized, double-blind controlled trial called the *Dalhousie Project.* In the *level I evidence experimental phase,* we injected both hands of 18 Dalhousie University alumnus hand surgeons who volunteered to have both their ring fingers injected in three sites with 1.8 ml of 2% lidocaine with epinephrine 1:100,000.[2] One hour later, we injected each of the three sites of one hand with 1 mg (1 ml) of phentolamine, and the three sites on the other hand were injected with 1 ml of saline solution. In the figure you can see the "phentolamine blush," where redness is returning around the three phentolamine injection sites one hour after we injected phentolamine in the left hand. The conclusion was that it took an average of 85 minutes for epinephrine-injected fingers to return to normal color after phentolamine injection, whereas it took an average of 320 minutes for epinephrine-injected fingers to return to normal color after injection of saline solution (no phentolamine).

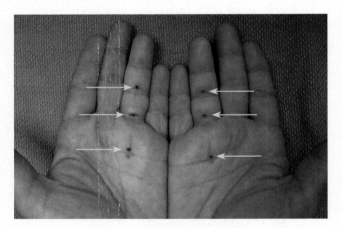

Phentolamine reversal of vasoconstriction after injection of 2% lidocaine with epinephrine 1:100,000. In the left hand, the arrows indicate that 2 ml of lidocaine and epinephrine only were injected. In the right hand, the arrows indicate lidocaine and epinephrine were injected, and 1 hour later, phentolamine was injected (1 mg in 1 ml).

MANAGING THE WHITE FINGERTIP

- Although finger infarction is rare, there is one reported case in which epinephrine with lidocaine may have played a partial role in a finger loss.[13]

- Most white fingertips will resolve without any treatment. However, to be on the safe side, you can reverse the white fingertip by injecting phentolamine wherever you have injected epinephrine before the patient leaves your facility.

- When you inject lidocaine with 1:100,000 epinephrine in the proximal or middle phalanx subcutaneous fat, those areas will go white, but the fingertip or thumb tip will usually remain pink.

- If you inject the local anesthetic into the sheath instead of the subcutaneous fat, it diffuses to the distal phalanx, where it has a greater chance of making the fingertip white. Local anesthetic injected into the sheath hurts more than local anesthetic injected into the subcutaneous fat.

TREATMENT OF ACCIDENTAL INJECTION OF HIGH-DOSE (1:1000) EPINEPHRINE IN THE FINGER

- Accidental injection of high-dose epinephrine occurs when people attempt to self-administer EpiPen or Ana-Kit injections to treat anaphylaxis in situations such as bee stings. Even though most of these individuals did not receive phentolamine rescue, in the hundreds of cases in the literature, there has been no reported finger loss.[5,14]

- You should treat these cases with phentolamine to prevent ischemic neurapraxia and ischemic reperfusion pain, which can both occur when it takes 14 hours for a finger to pink up.[6] The dosage to reverse epinephrine vasoconstriction in the finger is to inject 1 mg of phentolamine in 1 ml or more of saline solution into the subcutaneous fat wherever there is severe epinephrine pallor in the skin.

References

1. Denkler K. A comprehensive review of epinephrine in the finger: to do or not to do. Plast Reconstr Surg 108:114, 2001.
2. Nodwell T, Lalonde DH. How long does it take phentolamine to reverse adrenaline-induced vasoconstriction in the finger and hand? A prospective randomized blinded study: the Dalhousie project experimental phase. Can J Plast Surg 11:187, 2003.
3. Lalonde DH, Bell M, Benoit P, Sparkes G, Denkler K, Chang P. A multicenter prospective study of 3,110 consecutive cases of elective epinephrine use in the fingers and hand: the Dalhousie Project clinical phase. J Hand Surg Am 30:1061, 2005.
4. Chowdhry S, Seidenstricker L, Cooney DS, Hazani R, Wilhelmi BJ. Do not use epinephrine in digital blocks: myth or truth? Part II. A retrospective review of 1111 cases. Plast Reconstr Surg 126:2031, 2010.

5. Fitzcharles-Bowe C, Denkler K, Lalonde D. Finger injection with high-dose (1:1,000) epi-nephrine: does it cause finger necrosis and should it be treated? Hand (N Y) 2:5, 2007.
6. Muck AE, Bebarta VS, Borys DJ, Morgan DL. Six years of epinephrine digital injections: absence of significant local or systemic effects. Ann Emerg Med 56:270, 2010.
7. Thomson CJ, Lalonde DH, Denkler KA, Feicht AJ. A critical look at the evidence for and against elective epinephrine use in the finger. Plast Reconstr Surg 119:260, 2007.
8. Uri J, Adler P. The disintegration of procaine solutions. Curr Res Anesth Analg 29:229, 1950.
9. Hydrolysis of procaine in aqueous buffer solutions. Acta Pharmacol 5:353, 1949.
10. Health Sciences Institute drug expiration dates. Available at *http://hsionline.com/2004/08/26/drug-expiration-dates-2/.*
11. Food and Drug Administration. Warning—procaine solution. JAMA 138:599, 1948.
12. Phentolamine description. Available at *http://www.drugs.com/pro/phentolamine.html.*
13. Ruiter T, Harter T, Miladore N, Neafus A, Kasdan M. Finger amputation after injection with lidocaine and epinephrine. Eplasty 14:ic43, 2014.
14. Muck AE, Bebarta VS, Borys DJ, Morgan DL. Six years of epinephrine digital injections: absence of significant local or systemic effects. Ann Emerg Med 56:270, 2010.

Chapter 4
Tumescent Local Anesthesia

Donald H. Lalonde, Alistair Phillips, Duncan McGrouther

Tumescent local anesthesia means injecting a large enough volume of local anesthetic that you can see it plump up the skin and feel its slightly firm consistency with your finger through the skin.

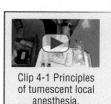

Clip 4-1 Principles of tumescent local anesthesia.

- Tumescent local anesthesia is like an extravascular Bier block, but the anesthetic is placed only where you need it. This technique avoids the risk associated with intravascular injection and the pain of a tourniquet.

- Always inject from proximal to distal so you are blocking nerves at the beginning of the injection process.

- Never elicit paresthesia with the needle. The presence of paresthesia means that you may have lacerated nerve fascicles. If you inject tumescent local anesthetic near any nerve, it will numb if given time. The larger the nerve, the longer it takes for anesthesia to peak. Our yet-unpublished studies have shown that median nerve anesthesia continues to increase 45 minutes after injection of tumescent local anesthetic.

- Local anesthetic will not impair visibility, because it is as clear as water. In fact, tumescent local anesthetic hydrodissects the tissue planes for the surgeon and facilitates the dissection.

- You can inject large areas such as the whole forearm and wrist with tumescent anesthetic in such a way that the patient only feels the first sting of a 27-gauge needle if you follow the simple guidelines presented in Chapter 5. Patients are amazed and delighted that the injection discomfort is minimal.

- You can also inject large areas with tumescent local anesthetic much more quickly with less bruising and minimal pain using blunt-tipped cannula needles (see more on cannula injection in Chapter 5).

- The use of tumescent local anesthetic injection with no tourniquet also helps significantly in cases requiring general anesthesia. It will decrease the bleeding, reduce the narcotic requirements administered by the anesthesiologist, and avoid having to deal with let-down bleeding that would occur when you release a tourniquet. The tumescent solution is simply injected as soon as the patient is asleep. You can then go scrub, prep, and drape the patient, and complete other tasks while the epinephrine takes effect.

TOO MUCH VOLUME IS BETTER THAN NOT ENOUGH VOLUME OF LOCAL ANESTHETIC—EXCEPT IN THE FINGERS

- Patients never complain of being too numb, but we have all had patients say that they were not numb enough and that we were hurting them.

- Strive to *never* have patients ask for "top-ups" or additional local anesthetic because they feel pain during the surgery. This creates an unnecessary, unpleasant memory for the patient. It is a sign of improper planning of the injection; the usual cause is not enough volume, with anesthetic not distributed widely enough.

- If you stay within safe limits of the total dosage of lidocaine and epinephrine, erring on the side of too much volume will eliminate the risk of requiring a top-up additional injection of local anesthetic because the patient reports feeling pain during an operation.

- The only exception to the rule of "too much local anesthetic is better than not enough" is in the fingers. No more than 2 ml of local anesthetic is required in each of the volar and dorsal sides of the proximal and middle phalanges of the fingers. Only 1 ml is required in the volar distal phalanx. If you inject too much volume of anesthetic in a finger, the pure compression effect of too much fluid can decrease blood flow. For nail bed work, a quarter-inch Penrose drain finger tourniquet works better than epinephrine injected in the dorsal distal phalanx.

- Always have at least 1 cm of visible or palpable subcutaneous local anesthetic beyond the site where you plan to incise, dissect, insert sutures, manipulate fractures, or pass K-wires.
  - Do not cut or insert needles where the skin is pink. Never reinsert a local anesthetic needle where the skin is not solidly white when you reinsert needles to inject large areas. If there are not enough epinephrine molecules there to produce good vasoconstriction, there will likely not be enough functioning lidocaine molecules there either. The patient will feel the needles and scalpels in the pinkish skin.
  - It is ideal to give the local anesthetic 30 minutes or more to work. It takes an average of 26 minutes for maximal cutaneous vasoconstriction to occur with 1:100,000 epinephrine.[1] It takes a similar amount of time for maximal numbness to occur with lidocaine. If you inject the patient in the recovery room or on a stretcher outside the operating room, the anesthetic will have time to work by the time you prep and drape the patient on the operating table.
  - For short procedures, inject the first three patients and do the paperwork before you operate on the first patient. After you operate on the first one, inject the fourth patient while the nurse brings the second injected patient into the room (see Chapter 14).
  - If your situation does not permit half an hour for the tumescent anesthetic to take effect, hemostasis is usually reasonable at 15 minutes after injection. The site will bleed a little more, but only an acceptably small amount.

IF YOU ARE WORKING WITH AN ANESTHESIOLOGIST

• Ask him or her to use only propofol. Inject the lidocaine with epinephrine as soon as the propofol permits pain-free injection of local anesthetic. The anesthesiologist can then wake the patient right away while you are scrubbing, prepping, and draping. This means you will have the benefit of an alert patient intraoperatively who can understand your teaching (see Chapter 8) and be fully cooperative with pain-free movement. This will also give the epinephrine a little time to become more effective. Suggest that the anesthesia provider avoid administering opiates and amnestics to prevent nausea and allow the patient to remember your intraoperative advice.

SAFE DOSAGE OF LIDOCAINE WITH EPINEPHRINE

• The widely quoted maximal dose of lidocaine with epinephrine is 7 mg/kg. This number originated before 1950, at the dawn of lidocaine use. Since then, Vasconez and others have reported safe blood levels of lidocaine when they injected 35 mg/kg for liposuction.[2,3]

• Because we do not monitor most of our patients, we stay within the very safe dose of 7 mg/kg, which is all we need to perform most hand operations. In a 70 kg adult, this means the following:

7 mg/kg × 70 kg = 490 mg or 49 ml of 1% lidocaine
with 1:100,000 epinephrine

Table 4-1 Safe Dosage for an Average Adult

Volume Needed (ml)	
<50	We use commercially available 1% lidocaine with 1:100,000 epinephrine (always buffered with 10 ml local anesthetic to 1 ml of 8.4% sodium bicarbonate to decrease the pain of injection[4]).
50-100	We dilute buffered 50 ml of commercially available 1% lidocaine with 1:100,000 epinephrine with 50 ml of saline solution to produce 100 ml of 0.5% lidocaine with 1:200,000 epinephrine.
100-200	We dilute buffered 50 ml of commercially available 1% lidocaine with 1:100,000 epinephrine with 150 ml of saline solution to produce 200 ml of 0.25% lidocaine with 1:400,000 epinephrine, which is clinically very effective both for local anesthesia and for vasoconstriction. The lower concentration just takes longer to work and does not last as long.

- In the average adult:
  - If we need less than 50 ml of volume, we use commercially available 1% lidocaine with 1:100,000 epinephrine (always buffered with 10 ml local anesthetic to 1 ml of 8.4% sodium bicarbonate to decrease the pain of injection[4]).
  - If we need 50 to 100 ml of volume, we dilute buffered 50 ml of commercially available 1% lidocaine with 1:100,000 epinephrine with 50 ml of saline solution to get 100 ml of 0.5% lidocaine with 1:200,000 epinephrine.
  - If we need 100 to 200 ml of volume, we dilute buffered 50 ml of commercially available 1% lidocaine with 1:100,000 epinephrine with 150 ml of saline solution to get 200 ml of 0.25% lidocaine with 1:400,000 epinephrine, which is clinically very effective both for local anesthesia and for vasoconstriction. The lower concentration just takes longer to work and does not last as long.

- You can finish most hand operations in the anesthesia time provided by lidocaine with epinephrine (5 hours in the wrist,[5] 10 hours in the finger[6]). We only use bupivacaine in operations that may last more than 2½ to 3 hours. We add 10 ml of 0.5% bupivacaine with 1:200,000 epinephrine to the total injection mixture in these cases.

THE GREATER THE CONCENTRATION OF EPINEPHRINE, THE LONGER AND MORE INTENSE THE VASOCONSTRICTION

One investigator had three fingers simultaneously injected with 0.5 ml of different concentrations of epinephrine in three fingers.[1] The small finger (injected with epinephrine 1:100,000) pinked up completely after 6 hours. It took 10 hours for vasoconstriction to reverse in the ring finger after injection of 1:10,000 epinephrine. The long finger took 14 hours for the pink color to completely return after injection of 1:1000 epinephrine.

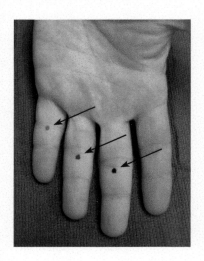

- Some surgeons use 1:1,000,000 epinephrine for WALANT[7] with good clinical results, but the epinephrine may not last as long as the 1:100,000 or 1:200,000 that most surgeons use.

- The designation 1:100,000 epinephrine means 1 g (1,000,000 µg) of epinephrine in 100,000 ml of saline solution, or 10 µg/ml.

- The designation 1:200,000 epinephrine means 1 g (1,000,000 µg) of epinephrine in 200,000 ml of saline solution, or 5 µg/ml.

DIFFERENT CONCENTRATIONS OF EPINEPHRINE PREMIXED WITH LIDOCAINE IN DIFFERENT COUNTRIES

- In Canada and the United States, the anesthetic comes premixed as 1% lidocaine with 1:100,000 epinephrine.

- At this writing, 1% lidocaine with 1:200,000 epinephrine is available as a premixed solution with lidocaine in many European countries, and this works very well for those surgeons. In Israel, premixed lidocaine with epinephrine is not available, and surgeons have to mix their own. In Hong Kong and Brazil, premixed 2% lidocaine with 1:200,000 epinephrine is used. Egypt has premixed 2% lidocaine with 1:100,000 of epinephrine. Indonesia has 2% lidocaine with 1:80,000 epinephrine. Clearly, published evidence is not yet guiding the worldwide availability of a single optimal combination.

- You can mix lidocaine and epinephrine with saline solution in the small 50 or 100 ml bags that saline comes in. If you remove 10 ml of saline from a 50 ml bag and then add 40 ml of 1% lidocaine with 1:100,000 epinephrine, you now have 80 ml of 0.5% lidocaine with 1:200,000 epinephrine.

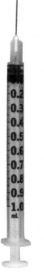
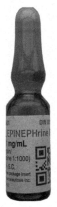

Another method (as recommended by Marco Felipe F.H. de Barros of Brazil) is to take one bottle of 20 ml of 2% plain lidocaine, add 0.4 ml of epinephrine 1:1000 (1 mg/ml), which produces 2% lidocaine with 1:50,000 epinephrine. You can mix 20 ml of this 2% lidocaine with 1:50,000 epinephrine with an equal volume of 20 ml of saline solution to produce 40 ml of 1% lidocaine with 1:100,000 epinephrine.

Insulin syringe   Epinephrine 1:1000

SCARS, CREASES, AND PALMAR/DORSAL BORDERS: THREE NATURAL BARRIERS TO DIFFUSION OF LOCAL ANESTHETIC SOLUTION

- Local anesthetic does not diffuse well across scars. You will most often need to inject local anesthetic on both sides of a linear scar, starting in unscarred healthy subcutaneous fat. For widely scarred areas, try to start proximal to distal injecting in healthy subcutaneous tissue all around the scarred area, then finishing under the scar if necessary.

- All skin creases in the hand and wrist, such as the crease between the fingers and palm, have ligaments that bind the skin to deeper structures, such as the flexor sheath. These can slow the diffusion of tumescent local anesthetic to the other side of the crease. Local anesthetic will cross below a skin crease, but only slowly and if under pressure with large volumes. It is wisest to inject on both sides of creases, starting from proximal to distal, to decrease the pain of injection.

- Where palmar glabrous skin meets dorsal nonglabrous skin, there are cutaneous ligaments that act as a third barrier to diffusion of local anesthesia. This zone is also a natural embryologic "largely nerve-free territory" line between the palm and dorsum of the hand, where the dorsal sensory system meets the palmar sensory system. It is a line where you can make incisions with less likelihood of neuroma formation.[8]

INFECTED HANDS

- In infected hands, injecting directly into inflamed tissues does not work very well because (1) it is painful, (2) the swollen tissues do not easily accept the extra local anesthetic volume, and (3) the hyperemia washes out lidocaine quickly, even with epinephrine.

- Instead of injecting into the infected area, inject tumescent local anesthetic first proximally and then around the affected site, and accept the fact that a little more bleeding will occur.

- In the clinic or emergency department in countries that regulate water cleanliness, you can wash a numbed infected draining hand in the sink, where a faucet delivers large volumes of clean water to wash out the pus from the wound (see Chapter 2). This also avoids contaminating clean main operating room theaters with pus.

PERSPECTIVE ON LOCAL ANESTHESIA

Duncan McGrouther

- My personal approach to administration of local anesthetic in the hand is to apply our knowledge of anatomy to capitalize on the gliding planes around the digital nerves. In former times, my personal success with axillary and supraclavicular nerve blocks was always less than 100%, with a frequent need to convert to general anesthesia. I have moved toward using local anesthetic with epinephrine injected directly into the hand.

- At the wrist, I have always had concerns about all injections, because there are many different planes and compartments where the needle may land. There is a potential risk of damaging a nerve fascicle, which can lead to ongoing symptoms of pain or paresthesias. For anesthesia of the proximal palm, I tend to inject proximal to the carpal canal, about 4 cm above the proximal wrist crease and through the deep fascia, where nerves are more mobile and damage is less likely. You can augment this later by direct subcutaneous injection of the lignocaine (lidocaine)/epinephrine mix in the palmar tissues to produce a dry operative field.

References

1. McKee DE, Lalonde DH, Thoma A, Glennie DL, Hayward JE. Optimal time delay between epinephrine injection and incision to minimize bleeding. Plast Reconstr Surg 131:811, 2013.
2. Burk RW III, Guzman-Stein G, Vasconez LO. Lidocaine and epinephrine levels in tumescent technique liposuction. Plast Reconstr Surg 97:1379, 1996.
3. Klein JA. Tumescent technique for regional anesthesia permits lidocaine doses of 35 mg/kg for liposuction. J Dermatol Surg Oncol 16:248, 1990.
4. Frank SG, Lalonde DH. How acidic is the lidocaine we are injecting, and how much bicarbonate should we add? Can J Plast Surg 20:71, 2012.
5. Chandran GJ, Chung B, Lalonde J, Lalonde DH. The hyperthermic effect of a distal volar forearm nerve block: a possible treatment of acute digital frostbite injuries? Plast Reconstr Surg 126:946, 2010.
6. Thomson CJ, Lalonde DH. Randomized double-blind comparison of duration of anesthesia among three commonly used agents in digital nerve block. Plast Reconstr Surg 118:429, 2006.
7. Prasetyono TO, Biben JA. "One-per-mil" tumescent technique for hand surgery. Plast Reconstr Surg 132:1091e, 2013.
8. Ritchie J. A comparison of trapeziectomy via anterior and posterior approaches. J Hand Surg Eur 33:137, 2008.

CHAPTER 5

HOW TO INJECT LOCAL ANESTHETIC WITH MINIMAL PAIN

Donald H. Lalonde, Nik Jagodzinski, Alistair Phillips

LOCAL ANESTHESIA DOES NOT HAVE TO HURT

We easily teach all of our medical students and residents how to inject local anesthetic for carpal tunnel surgery so that all the patient consistently feels is the first stick of a 27- or 30-gauge needle.[1] Patients will greatly appreciate the doctor who has invested the time required to learn the ten simple rules listed below.[2] *The most important are rules 7, 8, 9, and 10.* Our patients are constantly amazed and delighted at how little pain they feel from our medical students' and residents' injections.

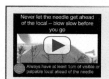

Clip 5-1 How to inject local anesthetic with minimal pain.

Clip 5-2 Patient's pain impressions after a "hole-in-one" local anesthetic injection for carpal tunnel surgery.

RULE 1. BUFFER 1% LIDOCAINE AND 1:100,000 EPINEPHRINE WITH 10:1 8.4% SODIUM BICARBONATE

- 1% lidocaine with 1:100,000 epinephrine has an average pH of 4.2, with a range of 3.3 to 5.5.[3] This can be 1000 times more acidic than the normal body pH of 7.4. This is one reason that it hurts when you inject it unbuffered.

- A bottle of 50 ml of 8.4% sodium bicarbonate costs less than $10.

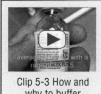

Clip 5-3 How and why to buffer lidocaine with epinephrine.

Conveniently, a 10 ml syringe actually holds 11 ml, and a 20 ml syringe holds 22 ml. Simply add 1 ml of 8.4% bicarbonate to 10 ml of 1% lidocaine and 1:100,000 epinephrine to make the pH body neutral.[1] Draw up 1 ml of sodium bicarbonate, then fill the rest of the 10 ml syringe to 11 ml with 1% lidocaine with 1:100,000 epinephrine. (From Strazar AR, Leynes PG, Lalonde DH. Minimizing the pain of local anesthesia injection. Plast Reconstr Surg 132:675, 2013.)

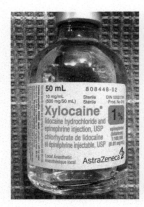
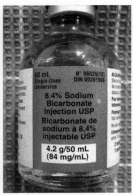

RULE 2. DO NOT USE REFRIGERATED LOCAL ANESTHETIC

• Refrigerated local anesthetic will result in a more uncomfortable injection for the patient than room-temperature local anesthetic.[4] We store our lidocaine with epinephrine at room temperature. Some centers keep their lidocaine and epinephrine refrigerated so that it lasts longer. This is not necessary if you simply adhere to the expiration dates on the bottle.

RULE 3. INJECT LOCAL ANESTHESIA WITH SMALL-BORE 27- OR 30-GAUGE NEEDLES

• Bigger needles hurt more. Stop using 25-gauge or larger needles.

• Injecting large volumes quickly causes pressure pain. Use smaller 27-gauge needles, which will remind you to slow down, which will decrease injection pain.

• Use 30-gauge needles for children or patients who are particularly sensitive.

RULE 4. CREATE SENSORY NOISE IN THE AREA OF INJECTION

• Simply pressing firmly on the skin proximal to where you will insert the needle can create sensory input "noise" that decreases the pain felt by the patient. This is like hearing a baby cry in a crowd versus hearing it cry in your room at 2 AM.

• It may hurt the patient more if he or she watches the needle go in.[5] Ask the patient to look away.

- Icing the skin[6] or vibrating it[7] can decrease the pain of needle entry.
- You can also move loose skin into the needle tip instead of moving the needle into the skin.

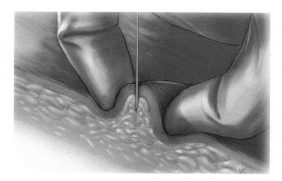

If the skin is loose, it can be gently pinched in the area into which the fine needle will be inserted. You can also move loose skin into the needle tip instead of moving the needle into the skin. These maneuvers provide sensory noise distraction, which decreases pain. (From Strazar AR, Leynes PG, Lalonde DH. Minimizing the pain of local anesthesia injection. Plast Reconstr Surg 132:675, 2013.)

RULE 5. STABILIZE THE SYRINGE WITH BOTH HANDS AND HAVE YOUR THUMB READY ON THE PLUNGER TO AVOID THE PAIN OF A MOVING NEEDLE

- It can take up to a minute for the needle site to numb after you place the needle under the skin, especially if you inject an insufficient bleb right under the dermis. In this time, the patient will feel the sting with every little wobble of the needle moving in the skin.
- If you stabilize the syringe with two hands, and if your thumb is on the plunger ready to inject before the needle penetrates, you will minimize painful needle movement in unanesthetized skin.

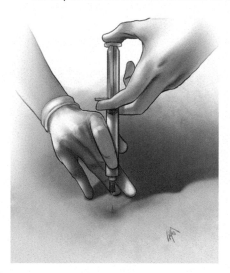

Stabilize the needle so it does not wobble until the skin is numb. Hold it with two hands. If the syringe-holding hand is free and is not stabilized on the skin, the patient will feel every little needle movement until the local anesthetic has numbed the needle insertion site. (From Strazar AR, Leynes PG, Lalonde DH. Minimizing the pain of local anesthesia injection. Plast Reconstr Surg 132:675, 2013.)

RULE 6. INJECT 0.5 ML WITH A PERPENDICULAR NEEDLE JUST UNDER THE DERMIS AND THEN PAUSE UNTIL THE PATIENT SAYS THE NEEDLE PAIN IS GONE

- Nerves in the dermis are like trees with sensitive leaves, and in the fat are like branches and trunks. Injections in the dermis hurt more than in subcutaneous fat, because you irritate more "leaves" with the pressure of intradermal injection.[8] Inject just under the dermis instead of in the dermis.

- Inserting the needle perpendicular (90 degrees) to the skin hurts less than if you come in parallel to it, because you pierce fewer nerve endings with the sharp needle tip on the way to the subcutaneous fat.[9]

- Begin by injecting a visible bleb (0.5 ml) just under the dermis, then pause until the patient tells you the pain is all gone. You will be able to start to count the number of subsequent times the patient feels pain. You can then score yourself as per rule 9 and improve your injection technique, because you will be able to count the total number of times the patient feels pain during the injection process.

- When the patient tells you the sting of the needle site is gone, inject an additional 1.5 ml very slowly without moving the needle.

- If you start to inject quickly or move the needle tip out of the numb zone, the patient will feel pain. After you have injected the initial 2 ml of anesthetic, you can change the angle from 90 perpendicular degrees to parallel to the skin without causing pain.

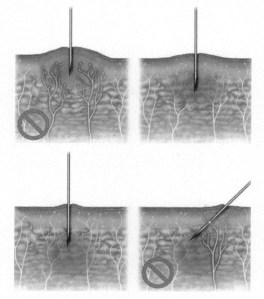

As soon as the needle is inserted, *blow in a visible bleb of 0.5 ml under the dermis, not in the dermis.* The needle should be inserted at 90 degrees so that fewer nerves are pierced. At a 90-degree angle, the patient will feel less pain than if the needle is inserted at a 45-degree angle. (From Strazar AR, Leynes PG, Lalonde DH. Minimizing the pain of local anesthesia injection. Plast Reconstr Surg 132:675, 2013.)

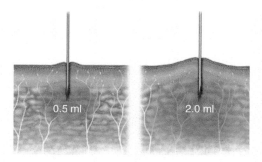

After you have injected 0.5 ml in the subcutaneous fat, hold still at least 15 seconds. Ask the patient to tell you when the sting of the needle is all gone. The first subcutaneous bleb or wheal must be visible or palpable under the skin in order for the needle insertion site to be properly numbed. After the patient tells you the sting of the needle is gone, inject an additional 1.5 ml very slowly without moving the needle. (From Strazar AR, Leynes PG, Lalonde DH. Minimizing the pain of local anesthesia injection. Plast Reconstr Surg 132:675, 2013.)

MOST IMPORTANT RULES

RULE 7. NEVER LET THE NEEDLE GET AHEAD OF THE LOCAL ANESTHETIC AND "BLOW SLOW BEFORE YOU GO"

- Hitting live nerves with a sharp needle tip hurts! Never let your needle tip hit nerves that are not numbed.

- Instead, blow slow before you go.

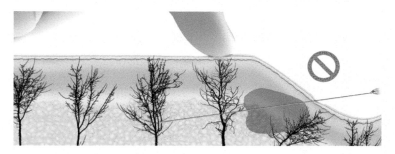

Never let the needle get ahead of the local anesthetic. If this happens, the sharp needle tip will irritate nerve endings that have not been numbed. Inject the local anesthetic in an antegrade fashion so the needle tip only enters numbed nerve territory. (From Strazar AR, Leynes PG, Lalonde DH. Minimizing the pain of local anesthesia injection. Plast Reconstr Surg 132:675, 2013.)

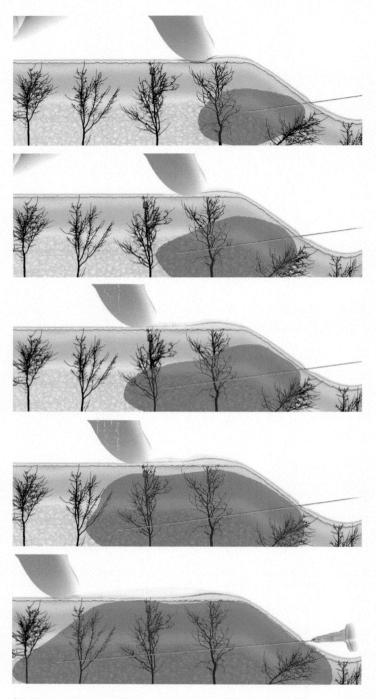

Always repeat the phrase "blow slow before you go" in your head while you are injecting. It will help you to slow down and be patient. If you inject in an antegrade direction while advancing very slowly and steadily under the skin, the sharp needle tip will only enter numbed territory. There should always be at least 1 cm of visible or palpable local anesthetic ahead of the sharp needle tip. (From Strazar AR, Leynes PG, Lalonde DH. Minimizing the pain of local anesthesia injection. Plast Reconstr Surg 132:675, 2013.)

RULE 8. REINSERT NEEDLES WITHIN 1 CM OF THE BLANCHED/UNBLANCHED BORDER

- Never reinsert the needle into unblanched skin. If there are not enough epinephrine molecules working there to cause vasoconstriction, chances are there is not enough lidocaine there for pain-free needle reinsertion.

- When you are injecting a large area (extensor indicis to extensor pollicis longus tendon transfer, for example), and you need to reinsert the injecting needle, reinsert the needle only into clearly blanched areas that are tumesced with visible or palpable local anesthetic (slightly firm to palpation). You should reinsert the needle 1 cm inside well-blanched skin beyond the border of the blanched/unblanched skin junction.

RULE 9. LEARN FROM EACH PATIENT YOU INJECT BY ASKING HIM OR HER TO GIVE YOU A SCORE

- Ask each patient to score you every time you inject local anesthetic. We have our patients score us and all our medical students and residents every time we inject so we can see that our scores continue to improve.

- Before you begin, ask the patient to tell you each time he or she feels pain during the injection process.

- If the patient does feel additional pain during the injection, stop moving the needle or back up a little and very, very slowly continue to inject in that one place until the pain is completely gone.
  - If the patient only feels the sting of the first needle stick, your pain score is 1 (hole-in-one).
  - If he or she feels pain a second time during the injection process, your pain score drops to 2 (eagle).
  - If the patient feels pain three times, you score a birdie, four times a bogie, and so on.

- Each patient you inject presents an opportunity for you to get better and better at injection. Each time we do not ask the patient to score us is a wasted opportunity to improve our technique.

- The most common reason that medical students and residents do not score a hole-in-one while injecting for carpal tunnel surgery is that they inject too quickly.[1] It takes about 5 minutes to consistently score a hole-in-one for carpal tunnel injection.

- *The three most common causes of poor pain scores are (1) injecting too quickly, (2) letting the sharp needle tip get ahead of the local anesthetic into unanesthetized areas, and (3) reinserting needles into "live," unanesthetized skin.*

RULE 10. TOO MUCH LOCAL ANESTHETIC IS BETTER THAN NOT ENOUGH LOCAL ANESTHETIC

- The more volume that you inject, the greater are the odds that the patient will feel no pain after you start to dissect. Try to avoid "top-ups" of local anesthetic that give patients unnecessary bad memories. Your patients do not want to feel pain during surgery any more than they want to wake up during a procedure in which they have been given a general anesthetic.

- Patients seldom complain about being too numb but frequently complain about not being numb enough. Stay within safe limits but always provide a little more volume than you need, except for the fingers, where you need only 2 ml per phalanx per side in the proximal and middle phalanges.

- *The two most common causes of needing a "top-up" are (1) not injecting enough volume of tumescent local anesthetic and (2) not giving the local anesthetic enough time to work (wait half an hour).*

OTHER DETAILS OF SHARP NEEDLE INJECTION

- Always inject from proximal to distal to anesthetize nerves proximally. The tumescent local anesthetic will create nerve blocks proximally.

- If you are blocking a major nerve as part of tumescent local anesthesia, never elicit paresthesias! If you do, you may have lacerated the nerve with your needle. Remember that a 25-gauge needle is the width of a human fascicle. You want to get near the nerve and inject a large volume to make certain you surround the nerve with local anesthetic.

- You may want to stage your injections for more time efficiency. For example, start by injecting 10 ml in the palm. This blocks the digital nerves of the fingers of interest. See or inject other patients while this takes effect. Come back 30 minutes later to perform all your distal injections quickly in the distal palm and fingers now that the nerve blocks have worked.

- Don't inject directly into a scar or skin crease. Scarred skin is tender and does not distend easily with local anesthetic. Skin creases exist because structures such as the tendon sheath adhere to the skin at that point with cutaneous ligaments, which are accompanied by sensitive nerve branches that feel the sharp pain of needle insertion. See Chapter 4 for details of injecting creased and scarred skin.

NEW BLUNT CANNULA INJECTION OF LOCAL ANESTHETIC

- New technology lets you inject with blunt-tipped cannulas instead of sharp needles. They are more expensive (about $5 to $10), but definitely faster and less painful than sharp needle tips.[10]

- See the clip in Chapter 18 for 37 mm blunt-tipped 27-gauge cannula injection for carpal tunnel.

- See the clip in Chapter 19 for 57 mm blunt-tipped 22-gauge cannula injection of local anesthetic for cubital tunnel release.

- See Chapter 27 clip for 40 mm long blunt-tipped 25-gauge cannula in an injection site made with a 20-gauge needle for trapeziectomy.

- The blunt needle tip can push quickly with no pain past "live," unanesthetized nerves by gliding in the fat. Sharp needle tips pierce nerves and cause pain if the local anesthetic is not bathing the nerve well ahead of the needle tip and if the operator is not moving slowly enough to let the local anesthetic work before the needle tip reaches the nerves.

- You insert blunt-tipped cannulas into skin injection sites made with sharp needles with a bore of larger diameter than that of the cannula so the cannula enters the injection site opening easily. For example, you insert a 22-gauge (5.7 cm long) cannula into an injection site opening made with a 20- or 21-gauge needle in anesthetized skin.

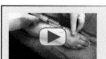

Clip 5-4 Cannula injection of tumescent local anesthetic for synovectomy and tendon transfer.

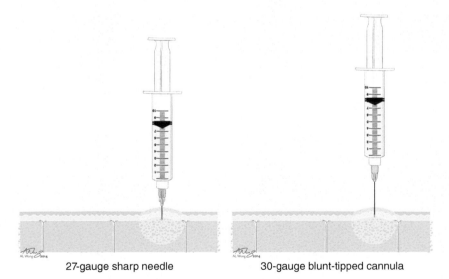

27-gauge sharp needle   30-gauge blunt-tipped cannula

First insert a minimally painful 27-gauge sharp needle just under the dermis, and inject 1 to 2 ml of buffered local anesthetic and create a hole for a 30-gauge blunt-tipped cannula insertion. Leave the inserting needle in the skin for a few seconds to stretch the cannulation entry hole to make it easier to find. Twirl the needle once or twice to help the hole stay open. Then insert a blunt-tipped 30-gauge cannula into the hole formed when you remove the sharp introducing 27-gauge needle. You sometimes need to patiently wait several seconds for the red blood dot to appear in the needle hole. Magnifying loupes are helpful to find the introducing needle hole. (From Lalonde D, Wong A. Local anesthetics: what's new in minimal pain injection and best evidence in pain control. Plast Reconstr Surg 134(Suppl 2):40S, 2014.)

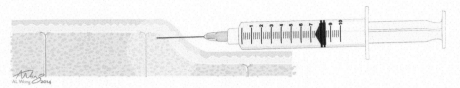

Inject the local anesthetic ahead of the blunt cannula tip as you advance it in the low-resistance fat. This remains painless as long as the injection rate is not too fast to cause pressure pain and as long as the cannula does not encounter resistance from cutaneous ligaments.

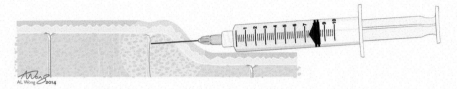

Pause the advance of the cannula when you encounter resistance. The cannula is probably butting up against a neurovascular bundle–ligament complex. Skin dimpling occurs at the area of resistance, and the patient may feel pain if that area is not numb. Inject solution at this barrier and then try backing up and finding an alternate resistance-free path into the fat instead of just pushing through the resisting tissue. Pushing through resistance areas that are not numb may be painful.

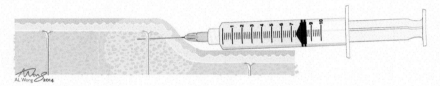

Redirect the cannula in a new path in resistance-free fat. When you encounter resistance, retreat the cannula and then advance at a different angle to find another path of minimal resistance through fat to avoid pain and bruising. (From Lalonde D, Wong A. Local anesthetics: what's new in minimal pain injection and best evidence in pain control. Plast Reconstr Surg 138(Suppl 2):40S, 2014.)

LEAST PAINFUL DIGITAL BLOCK: TWO DORSAL INJECTION BLOCK VERSUS SIMPLE BLOCK

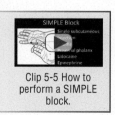

Clip 5-5 How to perform a SIMPLE block.

- The two dorsal injection block hurts more than the SIMPLE block, which stands for *s*ingle *s*ubcutaneous *i*njection in the *m*iddle of the *p*roximal *p*halanx with *l*idocaine and *e*pinephrine.[11,12]

- Injecting a SIMPLE block over 60 seconds hurts less than injecting it over 10 seconds.[13]

- Inject 2 ml of lidocaine and epinephrine in the fat just beneath the skin just past the palmar/digital crease between the two digital nerves.

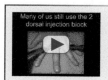

Clip 5-6 A two dorsal injection block hurts more than a SIMPLE block.

References

1. Farhangkhoee H, Lalonde J, Lalonde DH. Teaching medical students and residents how to inject local anesthesia almost painlessly. Can J Plast Surg 20:169, 2012.

2. Strazar AR, Leynes PG, Lalonde DH. Minimizing the pain of local anesthesia injection. Plast Reconstr Surg 132:675, 2013.

3. Frank SG, Lalonde DH. How acidic is the lidocaine we are injecting, and how much bicarbonate should we add? Can J Plast Surg 20:71, 2012.

4. Hogan ME, vanderVaart S, Perampaladas K, Machado M, Einarson TR, Taddio A. Systematic review and meta-analysis of the effect of warming local anesthetics on injection pain. Ann Emerg Med 58:86, 2011.

5. Höfle M, Hauck M, Engel AK, Senkowski D. Viewing a needle pricking a hand that you perceive as yours enhances unpleasantness of pain. Pain 153:1074, 2012.

6. Aminabadi NA, Farahani RM. The effect of pre-cooling the injection site on pediatric pain perception during the administration of local anesthesia. J Contemp Dent Pract 10:43, 2009.

7. Nanitsos E, Vartuli R, Forte A, Dennison PJ, Peck CC. The effect of vibration on pain during local anaesthesia injections. Aust Dent J 54:94, 2009.

8. Arndt KA, Burton C, Noe JM. Minimizing the pain of local anesthesia. Plast Reconstr Surg 72:676, 1983.

9. Martires KJ, Malbasa CL, Bordeaux JS. A randomized controlled crossover trial: lidocaine injected at a 90-degree angle causes less pain than lidocaine injected at a 45-degree angle. J Am Acad Dermatol 65:1231, 2011.

10. Lalonde D, Wong A. Local anesthetics: what's new in minimal pain injection and best evidence in pain control. Plast Reconstr Surg 134(4 Suppl 2):40S, 2014.

11. Williams JG, Lalonde DH. Randomized comparison of the single-injection volar subcutaneous block and the two-injection dorsal block for digital anesthesia. Plast Reconstr Surg 118:1195, 2006.

12. Wheelock ME, Leblanc M, Chung B, Williams J, Lalonde DH. Is it true that injecting palmar finger skin hurts more than dorsal skin? New level I evidence. Hand (N Y) 6:47, 2011.

13. Hamelin ND, St-Amand H, Lalonde DH, Harris PG, Brutus JP. Decreasing the pain of finger block injection: level II evidence. Hand (N Y) 8:69, 2013.

CHAPTER 6

DEALING WITH SYSTEMIC ADVERSE REACTIONS TO LIDOCAINE AND EPINEPHRINE

Donald H. Lalonde

THE SAFETY OF SYSTEMIC LIDOCAINE AND EPINEPHRINE INJECTION

- The only drugs required for most hand surgery procedures are lidocaine (also called lignocaine) and epinephrine.

- Lidocaine was introduced in the late 1940s, and in the intervening 65 years, American dentists have injected lidocaine premixed with epinephrine in an average of more than a million patients per day with no monitoring, no intravenous insertion, and no preoperative testing and have reported very few adverse reactions.[1,2] If there were common or serious problems with lidocaine and epinephrine injection, the American legal community would have been seeking financial compensation for their clients from dentists long ago.

- The maximal dose of lidocaine with epinephrine, published before 1950, is 7 mg/kg. Since then, Vasconez and others have reported safe blood levels of lidocaine when they injected 35 mg/kg for liposuction.[3,4]

- Lidocaine is much less cardiotoxic than other local anesthetics such as bupivacaine or ropivacaine (see the section on longer-lasting local anesthetics). In fact, internists commonly inject lidocaine to rescue ventricular arrhythmias.[5]

- A PubMed search for lidocaine anaphylaxis reveals six case reports in the past 7 years. Two of the six cases had incomplete details,[6,7] and the remaining four had other confounding variables, which made it hard to attribute the anaphylaxis solely to the lidocaine.[8-11] These reports are rare when you consider the billions of lidocaine doses administered in dental offices in the world in six and a half decades. If life-threatening anaphylaxis to lidocaine actually does exist, it is likely to be extremely rare.[12]

- Emergentologists inject lidocaine in 100 mg slow intravenous boluses to treat various pain conditions.[13] Anesthesiologists inject 1 mg/kg of lidocaine intravenously for pain control in postoperative patients.[14] Inadvertent intravenous small boluses of local anesthetic may occur with antegrade injection, as described in Chapter 4. However, toxicity from these tiny intravascular doses is very unlikely.

TREATMENT OF SYSTEMIC ADVERSE REACTIONS TO LIDOCAINE AND EPINEPHRINE

- Lidocaine-induced seizures can occur with large intravenous doses administered too quickly, or with excessive doses injected subcutaneously. With the doses and slow injection technique outlined in Chapters 4 and 5, this complication is likely to be rare or nonexistent. The treatment of lidocaine-induced seizures is conservative management.[15]

- The antidote for lidocaine toxicity is the lipid emulsion Intralipid. It has very limited use, because people rarely need it. It is not a perfect antidote.[16,17] The mechanism of action of lipid emulsion therapy for lidocaine toxicity is not well defined. It has been postulated that it works by a "lipid sink," decreasing circulating amounts of drugs to the periphery, or through a direct "energy source" to the myocardium.[5]

- The antidote of epinephrine vasoconstriction is phentolamine. The myth that epinephrine vasoconstriction is dangerous in fingers is addressed in Chapter 3. This chapter only deals with the systemic effects.

- The medical literature is almost devoid of reports of serious systemic adverse reactions to the epinephrine that accompanies the lidocaine, even in patients with cardiac disease.[18] However, if there is a concern about giving a patient with cardiac disease epinephrine-containing local anesthetic, we can monitor these patients and give them lower dosages of epinephrine.

- Clip 6-1 shows an 84-year-old man with cardiac issues who was given a lowered epinephrine concentration in the hospital with monitors during WALANT surgery for EI to EPL tendon transfer, with a good result.

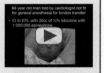

Clip 6-1 Lowered epinephrine concentration for cardiac issues.

- Epinephrine still provides good hemostasis in doses as low as 1:400,[19] or 1:1,000,000.[20] We routinely use 1:400,000 epinephrine when we need 100 to 200 ml of volume for larger cases and find the hemostasis perfectly acceptable, as long as we give the epinephrine half an hour to work.

- Epinephrine in a local anesthetic can cause transient elevation of the heart rate and blood pressure, but the clinical importance of this effect remains unclear.[5,21] Adverse outcomes among hypertensive patients are infrequent, and hemodynamic outcomes, which are possible risk indicators, reflect only minimal change.[17]

LONGER-LASTING LOCAL ANESTHETICS

- Ropivacaine and bupivacaine both last longer than lidocaine, but they have a lower safety profile. In large doses, bupivacaine[22,23] and ropivacaine[24,25] can be cardiotoxic and fatal. Lipid emulsion therapy has been used for both bupivacaine[26] and lidocaine[27] rescue.

- For digital blocks, bupivacaine-induced useful numbness to pain lasts only half as long (15 hours) as the annoying pressure and touch numbness (30 hours).[28] That is why patients with bupivacaine digital blocks complain that their injured finger is still numb, but it hurts.

- Lidocaine pain and numbness to touch and pressure all come back at the same time, like an on/off light switch.

- You can finish most hand operations in the anesthesia time provided by lidocaine with epinephrine (5 hours in the wrist,[29] 10 hours in the finger[30]). We use bupivacaine only in operations that may last more than 2½ to 3 hours or in procedures such as a trapeziectomy, where postoperative pain may be severe.

THE EPINEPHRINE "RUSH" AND THE VASOVAGAL ATTACK (FAINTING)

- Although lidocaine and epinephrine are probably two of the safest drugs in use, injecting them can have two relatively common adverse events. These are the epinephrine "rush" and the vasovagal attack in response to receiving a needle injection.

THE EPINEPHRINE RUSH

- About one third of patients can feel an epinephrine "rush," "jitter," "shakiness," "nervousness" or a feeling "like you have had too much coffee" for up to 20 to 30 minutes after an injection of local anesthetic.

- Forewarned is forearmed. We warn all of our patients that they may get this rushy feeling after we inject them. We tell them that this is not an allergy; it is a normal reaction to the epinephrine we have injected with the lidocaine, and the sensation will go away in 20 to 30 minutes.

- Catecho-o-methyl transferase and monoamine oxidase rapidly break down epinephrine in plasma[31] so that its half-life inside blood vessels is only 1.7 minutes.[32] However, extravascular epinephrine degradation is slower. The molecules must first get into blood vessels either by diffusion or through the lymphatics. You can frequently see white lymphatic vasoconstriction tracks in the forearm when you inject epinephrine into the hand.

AVOIDING THE FAINT

- Loss of consciousness that occurs with a faint or vasovagal attack occurs because there is not enough blood going to the brain. Nature's solution is to bring the head down by fainting to allow more blood to get to the brain with gravity (see the box on p. 52).

- A bandage change or cast removal can trigger fainting. Needles with or without local anesthetic are another common trigger.

Managing Fainting

Recognizing That Someone Is Going to Faint

Patients can faint even if you inject them lying down.

- The following are signs that a patient is about to faint. The patient may say "I'm not feeling well," or "I think I'm going to be sick (vomit)." If you look at the patient, he or she may be pale in the central upper face (glabella, between the eyes, upper nose, or perioral skin).

When a Faint Is Impending

If your patient is showing signs that he or she is about to faint, get more blood to the brain with the following gravity-changing maneuvers.

- Have the patient lie down if he or she is sitting. (We do not recommend anesthetic injection in the sitting position.)
- If the patient is lying down, put your hand beneath the knees and raise the knees up to flex the hips and knees so the thigh blood can run down toward the brain.
- Remove the pillow from under the head and place it under the feet.
- Lower the head of the stretcher to the Trendelenburg position (head down, feet up).

MANAGING THE FAINT

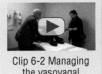

Clip 6-2 Managing
the vasovagal
fainting attack.

- If you inject patients in the lying-down position, fainting is less likely, because gravity causes more blood to get to the brain when the head is down.

- Raise the knees, place a pillow under the feet, and lower the stretcher to the Trendelenburg position.

THE ANXIOUS PATIENT

- Most anxious patients can be reassured with a quiet, soothing voice and manner. Most will tolerate wide awake hand surgery if they can tolerate a dental procedure.

- Music can be helpful to decrease anxiety.

- Some anxious patients do better with sedation. You can give them small oral doses of medication or provide full main operating room sedation with an anesthesiologist. The downside is that the patient will not be able to receive and remember intraoperative teaching and may not be able to help you by cooperatively moving the hand to assess its function during surgery.

References

1. Gaffen AS, Haas DA. Survey of local anesthetic use by Ontario dentists. J Can Dent Assoc 75:649, 2009.
2. Jeske AH. Xylocaine: 50 years of clinical service to dentistry. Tex Dent J 115:9, 1998.
3. Burk RW III, Guzman-Stein G, Vasconez LO. Lidocaine and epinephrine levels in tumescent technique liposuction. Plast Reconstr Surg 97:1379, 1996.
4. Klein JA. Tumescent technique for regional anesthesia permits lidocaine doses of 35 mg/kg for liposuction. J Dermatol Surg Oncol 16:248, 1990.
5. Dogru K, Duygulu F, Yildiz K, Kotanoglu MS, Madenoglu H, Boyaci A. Hemodynamic and blockade effects of high/low epinephrine doses during axillary brachial plexus blockade with lidocaine 1.5%: a randomized, double-blinded study. Reg Anesth Pain Med 28:401, 2003.
6. Al-Dosary K, Al-Qahtani A, Alangari A. Anaphylaxis to lidocaine with tolerance to articaine in a 12 year old girl. Saudi Pharm J 22:280, 2014.
7. Khokhlov VD, Krut' MI, Sashko Slu. [Anaphylactic shock following administration of lidocaine after negative skin test] Klin Med (Mosk) 90:62, 2012.
8. Lee MY, Park KA, Yeo SJ, Kim SH, Goong HJ, Jang AS, Park CS. Bronchospasm and anaphylactic shock following lidocaine aerosol inhalation in a patient with butane inhalation lung injury. Allergy Asthma Immunol Res 3:280, 2011.
9. Soong WJ, Lee YS, Soong YH, Yang CF, Jeng MJ, Peng YY. Life-threatening anaphylactic reaction after the administration of airway topical lidocaine. Pediatr Pulmonol 46:505, 2011.
10. Sinha M, Sinha R. Anaphylactic shock following intraurethral lidocaine administration during transurethral resection of the prostate. Indian J Urol 24:114, 2008.
11. Culp JA, Palis RI, Castells MC, Lucas SR, Borish L. Perioperative anaphylaxis in a 44-year-old man. Allergy Asthma Proc 28:602, 2007.
12. Specjalski K, Kita-Milczarska K, Jassem E. The negative predictive value of typing safe local anesthetics. Int Arch Allergy Immunol 162:86, 2013.
13. Tanen DA, Shimada M, Danish DC, Dos Santos F, Makela M, Riffenburgh RH. Intravenous lidocaine for the emergency department treatment of acute radicular low back pain, a randomized controlled trial. J Emerg Med 47:119, 2014.
14. Barreveld A, Witte J, Chahal H, Durieux ME, Strichartz G. Preventive analgesia by local anesthetics: the reduction of postoperative pain by peripheral nerve blocks and intravenous drugs. Anesth Analg 116:1141, 2013.
15. Aminiahidashti H, Laali A, Nosrati N, Jahani F. Recurrent seizures after lidocaine ingestion. J Adv Pharm Technol Res 6:35, 2015.
16. Heinonen JA, Litonius E, Salmi T, Haasio J, Tarkkila P, Backman JT, Rosenberg PH. Intravenous lipid emulsion given to volunteers does not affect symptoms of lidocaine brain toxicity. Basic Clin Pharmacol Toxicol 116:378, 2015.
17. Agency for Healthcare Research and Quality. Cardiovascular effects of epinephrine in hypertensive dental patients. Summary, evidence report/technology assessment: Number 48. AHRQ Publication Number 02-E005. Rockville, MD: The Agency, Mar 2002. Available at *http://hstat.nlm.nih.gov/ftrs/directBrowse.pl?collect=epc&dbname=ephysum*.
18. Sanatkar M, Sadeghi M, Esmaeili N, Naseri MH, Sadrossadat H, Shoroughi M, Fathi HR, Ghazizadeh S. The evaluation of perioperative safety of local anesthesia with lidocaine containing epinephrine in patients with ischemic heart disease. Acta Med Iran 51:537, 2013.
19. Kämmerer PW, Krämer N, Esch J, Pfau H, Uhlemann U, Piehlmeier L, Daubländer M. Epinephrine-reduced articaine solution (1:400,000) in paediatric dentistry: a multicentre non-interventional clinical trial. Eur Arch Paediatr Dent 14:89, 2013.
20. Prasetyono TO, Biben JA. One-per-mil tumescent technique for upper extremity surgeries: broadening the indication. J Hand Surg Am 39:3, 2014.

21. Abu-Mostafa N, Aldawssary A, Assari A, Alnujaidy S, Almutlaq A. A prospective random-ized clinical trial compared the effect of various types of local anesthetics cartridges on hypertensive patients during dental extraction. J Clin Exp Dent 7:e84, 2015.

22. Dudley MH, Fleming SW, Garg U, Edwards JM. Fatality involving complications of bupi-vacaine toxicity and hypersensitivity reaction. J Forensic Sci 56:1376, 2011.

23. Cordell CL, Schubkegel T, Light TR, Ahmad F. Lipid infusion rescue for bupivacaine-induced cardiac arrest after axillary block. J Hand Surg Am 35:144, 2010.

24. Gnaho A, Eyrieux S, Gentili M. Cardiac arrest during an ultrasound-guided sciatic nerve block combined with nerve stimulation. Reg Anesth Pain Med 34:278, 2009.

25. Hübler M, Gäbler R, Ehm B, Oertel R, Gama de Abreu M, Koch T. Successful resuscita-tion following ropivacaine-induced systemic toxicity in a neonate. Anaesthesia 65:1137, 2010.

26. Harvey M, Cave G, Chanwai G, Nicholson T. Successful resuscitation from bupivacaine-induced cardiovascular collapse with intravenous lipid emulsion following femoral nerve block in an emergency department. Emerg Med Australas 23:209, 2011.

27. Dix SK, Rosner GF, Nayar M, Harris JJ, Guglin ME, Winterfield JR, Xiong Z, Mudge GH Jr. Intractable cardiac arrest due to lidocaine toxicity successfully resuscitated with lipid emulsion. Crit Care Med 39:872, 2011.

28. Calder K, Chung B, O'Brien C, Lalonde DH. Bupivacaine digital blocks: how long is the pain relief and temperature elevation? Plast Reconstr Surg 131:1098, 2013.

29. Chandran GJ, Chung B, Lalonde J, Lalonde DH. The hyperthermic effect of a distal volar forearm nerve block: a possible treatment of acute digital frostbite injuries? Plast Recon-str Surg 126:946, 2010.

30. Thomson CJ, Lalonde DH. Randomized double-blind comparison of duration of anes-thesia among three commonly used agents in digital nerve block. Plast Reconstr Surg 118:429, 2006.

31. Kopin IJ. Monoamine oxidase and catecholamine metabolism. J Neural Transm 41:57, 1994.

32. Rosen SG, Linares OA, Sanfield J, Zech LA, Lizzio VP, Halter JB. Epinephrine kinetics in humans: radiotracer methodology. J Clin Endocrinol Metab 69:753, 1989.

Chapter 7

Tips on Talking to Your Patients About WALANT

Nik Jagodzinski, Alistair Phillips, Donald H. Lalonde

MANAGING PATIENT EXPECTATIONS BEFORE SURGERY

- For patients, fear of the unknown and anxiety about pain are the two biggest concerns about being awake during hand surgery. However, if we explain the process to patients calmly, clearly, and with confidence, we can quell the fear of the unknown so that most patients are reassured. By gaining knowledge of the procedure, the patient can feel more like an active participant in the treatment process, awake and cooperating. If we inject local anesthetic thoughtfully, as described in Chapter 5, it really does make the local anesthetic injection and surgery pain free, except for the initial pinch with a 27-gauge needle. The patient will be amazed at how brief and minor the discomfort is.

THINGS TO TELL PATIENTS DURING THE CONSULTATION SO THEY UNDERSTAND THE PROCEDURE BETTER

- Wide awake surgery is as simple as when you go to the dentist for a filling. We put in the freezing/numbing medicine, we perform the surgery, and then you get up and go home. (When asked, most patients say that it is a more pleasant experience than going to the dentist.)

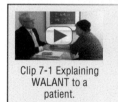

Clip 7-1 Explaining WALANT to a patient.

- You will not need to undergo any tests before surgery. That means you do not need to leave work or pay a babysitter to go for tests on a day before your surgery. You just need to arrive the day of surgery.

- You do not have to stop taking any medication before surgery.

- You do not have to fast before surgery or change any diabetic treatment routine.

- No intravenous line will be placed, so there will be no uncomfortable needle in your unoperated hand.

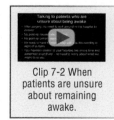

Clip 7-2 When patients are unsure about remaining awake.

- You will be amazed at how little the freezing/numbing medicine hurts when we put it in slowly with a tiny needle. Most people just feel one little needle prick in the hand, and then they feel no pain at all (see Chapter 5).

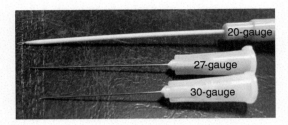

Comparison of the relative size of needles for sedation and wide awake hand surgery. The 20-gauge cannula is used for sedation; a 20-gauge needle is used for preoperative testing. The 27-gauge or 30-gauge needles are used for WALANT.

- The needle prick you will feel will be smaller than the sting of an intravenous insertion if we were using a general anesthetic, because we use a much smaller needle.

- *For those who are especially afraid of needles and therefore request sedation:* If you have sedation, you will have two needle sticks with bigger needles than the single prick you will feel if we numb you with a local anesthetic. You get two bigger needles if you want to be asleep: the first larger one is for blood tests, then you get another one with an intravenous line inserted to put you to sleep.

- In Clip 7-3 a patient describes the impression of pain of a local anesthetic needle for trapeziectomy versus the pain of intravenous needle insertion. This patient just had 40 ml of local anesthetic to numb up the radial hand, as described in Chapters 5 and 27.

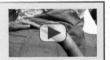

Clip 7-3 Patient impression of pain of a local anesthetic needle versus an intravenous needle.

- We will not be putting an uncomfortable tourniquet on your arm *(for those who have had experience with a tourniquet or have heard about it).*

- *For tendon or bone reconstruction:* You will be able to help me get a better result. After I fix your tendon, you can move it to make sure it is working properly. Sometimes I need to adjust what I have done, because your repaired tendon does not want to fit in the tunnel it lives in after I fix it. If you move your broken finger after I fix it, I can be sure that I have it straight. We are more likely to get a good result if you are awake to help me get it right. You cannot move it if you are asleep or sedated during the procedure.

- After the surgery, there is no need to wait around in the hospital to recover. You just get up and go home.

- You will not be nauseated and you will not vomit if you are not sedated.

- You will not have trouble urinating after surgery if you do not receive sedation.

- Staying awake is safer than sedation, because the safest sedation is no sedation. This is especially important for you because of your other medical problems [such as your lung problem . . .].

- You do not have to worry about what will happen to you. You can just ask us anything at any time before as well as during the procedure if you have concerns.

- You can watch if you wish. Many patients do enjoy watching parts of the surgery. Some tell their friends that watching the surgery should be on their "bucket list." However, you do not have to watch anything if you do not want to.

- You can bring headphones and listen to music during the surgery.

- It is very uncommon for anyone to feel pain during the surgery, but if you did, you would just tell me and I would add more local anesthetic.

- If you have a sore shoulder or back, let us know and we will help you adjust to a more comfortable position, such as on your side, during the surgery.

- Bring a book to read. After we inject the local anesthetic, you need to wait at least a half hour before we do the surgery. It is like putting a cake in the oven: you need to let it bake.

- You can ask me any questions during the surgery, and I will be happy to answer all of them.

- While I am operating, we can also discuss details about how you should care for your hand after the surgery.

- You do not need to get undressed (for patients for whom field sterility will be used, see Chapter 10). You will simply roll up your sleeve and have the surgery. You may want to wear short sleeves or a loose long-sleeve shirt so the bandage fits in easily.

- You will not need to have someone stay with you the evening of surgery, because you will not have had sedation. It will be safe for you to be alone with your children or elderly parents the evening of surgery. If you were to have sedation, the hospital would tell you that you need to have someone stay with you at home the evening of surgery.

THINGS TO TELL PATIENTS ABOUT THE DAY OF SURGERY

- You may be in the hospital 1 to 4 hours at most. (Add 1 hour to the surgery time to allow for a slow injection and half an hour to allow the local anesthetic to work.)

- You will have time to talk to me before and while we inject the local anesthetic. We inject it slowly so it will hurt less.

- Occasionally, people become faint when they get a needle. Has this ever happened to you? We numb people while they are lying down to avoid this. If you tend to faint, we will tilt the stretcher so your head is lower than your feet, and this will help to prevent your fainting.

- After we finish the injection, you may feel a bit jittery, as if you have had too much coffee, or like you are a little nervous. It is not your nerves. It's because there is a little adrenaline in the numbing medication, and these feelings are completely normal and not dangerous. If it does happen, the shaky feeling wears off all by itself in 5 to 30 minutes. It doesn't mean anything is wrong.

- You will then go back to the waiting room to give the numbing medicine time to work for at least a half an hour. You can read, talk to your friends, or listen to music.

- All you will feel is the cold and wet of us washing your hand and maybe a little pulling and tugging during the surgery.

- After the surgery, you will just get up and go home with your hand held higher than your heart. Your hand will be "on strike" for 2 or 3 days. We don't want you to move your fingers in that time so you do not bleed inside the wound. This will also allow the swelling to go away and will decrease your pain.

- Technically, you could drive a car because you did not get sedation. However, also technically, you are "impaired," since you will only have one normally functioning hand. Because you are not used to this situation, your driving may not be safe. If you were in an accident and it was your fault, it would be hard for you to justify in court that you were driving with one hand impaired, even if you were sedation free and pain free while the local anesthetic was still working.

CHAPTER 8

TALKING WITH PATIENTS DURING SURGERY SAVES TIME

Donald H. Lalonde, Duncan McGrouther

- During the years when we performed hand surgery with sedation, there was no point in educating patients during the surgery. They would not remember what we told them because of amnestic medications. With each passing year of wide awake hand surgery, it is becoming more and more apparent *that patient education during surgery is very helpful in many ways.* You can educate your patients about postoperative care and how to avoid complications while you are operating, and this is a better use of your time than chatting with the nurses about the weather.

- The time you spend talking to patients during the surgery is time you do not need to spend with them in the office before or after the surgery.

- Investing time to educate the patient during the surgery will save the time that would be lost on complications that occurred because the patient did not know how to look after his or hand postoperatively. Educated patients understand the importance of their rehabilitation protocols, are more likely to be compliant with postoperative instructions, and may require fewer follow-up appointments.

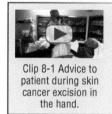

Clip 8-1 Advice to patient during skin cancer excision in the hand.

- You often find out important details about the patient's life and activities that you did not learn about in the initial consultation.

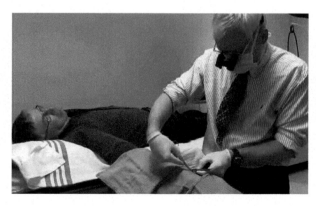

Talking to patients during surgery not only gives them something to think about and puts their minds at ease, but also provides them with information about all aspects of their problem, the likely course of recovery and rehabilitation, and gives you the opportunity to address any questions they may have.

- Patients love personal education in a nonrushed fashion from their surgeon. They are able to develop a one-on-one bond with you that was not possible in the days when sedation meant they had no memory of the procedure, and they did not feel that they were an active participant in the process.

- Patients know exactly what their hand should look like. If you have reduced a crooked finger, they can tell you if you have it right before you leave the operating room.

- Talking with patients during flexor tendon repair about how to look after their hand after surgery can decrease your rupture and tenolysis rates (see Chapter 32).

- Talking with patients during finger fracture repair about how to look after their hand after surgery can decrease your stiff finger rate.

- In Clip 8-3 advice is given to a patient, while the finger fracture is K-wired, about how to look after the finger in the days after surgery. Chapter 41 has a clip of this patient's whole care, including advice about early protected movement. Chapter 41 also has a clip on intraoperative advice for finger fracture patients.

- With complicated procedures such as a flexor tendon repair or a K-wired finger fracture, patients leave the operating room with a full understanding of how to take good care of their hand after surgery to get a better result. They understand that if they move the hand too much, the repair will fall apart. If they do not move it at all, everything will become stuck.

- A 10-year-old is given advice in Clip 8-4 during flexor tendon repair about how to look after the finger in the days after surgery. Chapter 9 has a clip of this patient's whole care.

- For a clip of a surgeon and therapist explaining the Saint John postoperative flexor tendon repair protocol to a patient during surgery, see Chapter 15.

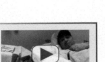

Clip 8-2 During surgery the patient can verify that the deformity has been corrected.

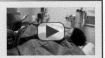

Clip 8-3 Advice to a patient while K-wiring a finger fracture.

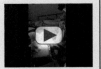

Clip 8-4 Advice to a 10-year-old during flexor tendon repair.

THINGS NOT TO SAY AND DO TO THE PATIENT DURING SURGERY

- Never say something like "Oops." Create an atmosphere of calm, efficiency, and competence.

- A silent surgeon can seem quite foreboding, while one who speaks too much without listening can also fail to reassure. The modern version of the "bedside manner" is the "operating table side manner."

- Do not ask the scrub nurse for a blade, scalpel, or skin hook. Use terms like "a number 15" and "single hook."

- Do not pass bloody swabs or instruments in front of the patient if you can avoid it.

EDUCATING TRAINEES TO PERFORM WALANT

- If you are teaching residents or medical students during the surgery, say things like "Well done! That was a perfect stitch," and so on. You may not normally be this complimentary to trainees, but patients are reassured when you like what the trainee is doing. This attitude goes a long way toward increasing patient confidence in the surgical teaching event.

- If you don't like what the resident is doing, nonverbal communication such as putting your hand between an instrument and his or her eyes is very effective.

- Say things such as "I know that some surgeons like to use the scissors this way when they do this part of the operation, but I like to use them this way, because . . ." as you take over the surgery.

- Softly saying, "Pause . . ." is also a good way to stop the action.

- This is clearly not the time or the place to reprimand a resident.

THINGS TO SAY TO PATIENTS WHEN YOU BEGIN THE INJECTION OF LOCAL ANESTHETIC

- It is good to begin with a calm, comfortable conversation about weather, family, or football before you inject the local anesthetic. Wait to focus on talking about the hand until the patient is as relaxed as possible.

- Your instructions to the patient should be polite and simply worded:
  - "Can you please lie down comfortably on your side? Would you kindly place your hand flat on the stretcher?"
  - "Try not to move when I put the needle in. If you pull away (which is normal when you get a little sting), the needle will come out before the medicine goes in, and I will need to put the needle in a second time. If you hold still, you will only feel one little stick instead of two. I will help you by holding your hand. OK? At the count of three, don't move. . . ."

- After you have started putting in the lidocaine and epinephrine, and the pain is completely gone (see Chapter 5), tell the patient it will take about 5 minutes for you to finish putting in the numbing medicine. "If I do it slowly, you will only feel the very first needle stick and that is all."

- As you inject the local anesthetic and have confirmed that the patient will no longer be feeling pain during the injection process, ask whether he or she has any questions about the surgery or about the care of the hand, when to go back to work, and other postsurgery issues. Take this 5-minute opportunity to answer questions and to tell the patient how to look after the hand after surgery.

THINGS TO TELL PATIENTS DURING CARPAL TUNNEL RELEASE (APPLICABLE TO MANY OPERATIONS)

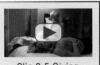

Clip 8-5 Giving intraoperative advice during carpal tunnel release.

- In Clip 8-5 a patient is given intraoperative advice during carpal tunnel release. This is also applicable to most other minor hand operations, such as trigger finger and flexor sheath ganglion. (See Chapter 18 for another clip on patient education during carpal tunnel release.)

- Instruct the patient: "Keep your hand higher than your heart for the next day or two. Consider that it is 'on strike.' Don't move your fingers or put your hand down until all of the numbing medicine is gone and until you are off all pain medications. If you keep your hand up and quiet, it will swell less, hurt less, and bleed less inside. Internal bleeding slows recovery. If you walk around with your hand dangling down, it will swell more, bleed more inside, hurt more, and stiffen more in the days to come."

- Ask patients what they usually take for pain. We tell them they can take up to 800 mg of Advil or Motrin (ibuprofen) and up to 1 g of Tylenol (acetaminophen) when the numbing medicine wears off. They can take ibuprofen and acetaminophen at the same time, because the two medications work in different ways.

- "There are two kinds of pain with any operation: (1) the pain of the incision, and (2) the pain of 'Gee, doctor, now it only hurts when I put my hand down or when I move.' The pain of the incision lasts a day or two, and you can take Advil or Tylenol for that pain. Stop taking pain medicine as soon as you get into the pain of 'Gee, doctor, now it only hurts when I put my hand down or when I move' and listen to your body. That pain is your friend. It is your body telling you, 'Hey there, I am not ready for that. I am trying to heal in here and you are screwing it up! Stop that!' That little voice inside your head is one that you should listen to."

- "We did not spend 2 billion years evolving pain because it is bad for us; it is our body's only way of telling us how to behave so we can heal faster."

- "You can remove your 'Hollywood' bandage (a 3-inch gauze roll so named because it is mostly applied for its visual effect) before you take a shower tomorrow. There is no problem with getting your wound wet in the shower. It's a myth that you can't wash fresh wounds; fresh wounds love running water. After the shower, you can gently pat the wound site dry with a towel. Put on a clean, dry Band-Aid and reuse or recycle the Hollywood bandage over the Band-Aid. The outer bandage does not need to be sterile, just clean. It is only there for visual effects to remind you and those around you that you can't do the things you normally do because you have had an operation. They will not shake your hand or ask you to do something that may hurt your hand. Stop using the outer bandage in 3 to 7 days. If your wound is dry and not oozing liquid any more, the germs cannot enter the wound, and no bandage is required. You may want to keep the bandage on for the Hollywood effect for sympathy or to protect yourself from small children and eager hand-shakers."

- "Don't baby your hand, but don't do anything that hurts. If you try to do something and it does hurt, don't try it again that afternoon. Do not try it again for 2 or 3 days. Healing takes days and weeks, not minutes and hours. You will get better faster if you listen to your body. It is very wise. It will tell you what you can and cannot do, but the only language it speaks is pain, and you may not be able hear it when you've taken Advil or Tylenol."

- "If you feel tingling or a small electrical shock sensation after surgery, this is normal. It is your body's natural healing mechanism at work. Your nerve is waking up after it has been compressed and asleep."

- "Redness on or around the incision is normal; redness less than the width of your thumb is healthy inflammation. The redness means that your body is bringing more blood to the wound edges to help with healing. Bruising in your forearm can also be normal. Infection is uncommon after a carpal tunnel procedure. Signs of infection include redness that goes all over your palm and up your forearm, with more and more pain in the incision instead of less and less pain, fever, chills, and real pus coming out of the wound (as opposed to a little clear liquid or blood in the first 2 or 3 days, which is normal)."

CHAPTER 9
WALANT HAND SURGERY IN INFANTS AND CHILDREN

Donald H. Lalonde

HOW TO EXPLAIN WALANT TO CHILDREN BEFORE YOU INJECT THE LOCAL ANESTHETIC

Children do very well with WALANT hand surgery. The key is to provide good local anesthesia (see Chapter 5) with a skillful injection so that all they feel is the first sting of a 30-gauge needle.

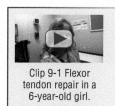

Clip 9-1 Flexor tendon repair in a 6-year-old girl.

- The most important factor in gaining the patient's trust and cooperation is how you talk to the child before you inject the local anesthetic. Using a calm, soft-spoken voice with a gentle manner and engaging conversation is very helpful. If you are not comfortable having a prolonged conversation with the child you are about to operate on, perhaps you should plan on performing the surgery with the patient under general anesthesia.

- The child must be old enough to understand your explanation and to hold still while you insert the first needle.

- If you can get the child to hold still to tolerate the stick of a 30-gauge needle in the finger or hand, you can perform the surgery with WALANT.

    The following approach works well with children: "Do you believe in magic?"

    Most children will say, "No."

    "Neither do I, but today I am going to show you some real magic. I am going to put some magic medicine underneath your skin. After I put it there, I will be able to fix your finger and it WILL NOT HURT AT ALL. I PROMISE YOU.

    The only problem with putting in the magic medicine is that you have to feel one tiny needle stick to get the medicine in there. All you need to do is hold still and not move.

    I will help you by holding your hand.

    If you pull your hand away before the medicine goes in, the needle will come out and I will have to stick it back in.

    If you hold still, you will only feel one little sting. If you move, you will feel two stings.

    Do you think you can hold still?"

- If the child gets that panicked look in the eyes that indicates he or she cannot hold still for the injection, general anesthesia is advisable.

- You need to keep your promise by making certain that all the child feels is the first sting, as shown in Chapter 5. Be sure that you have more than enough volume of anesthetic rather than not enough. Children should not have to have "top-ups."

- I usually have my body between the patient's eyes and her hands. Note that in Clip 9-2 my body is in an awkward position on the wrong side of the table for this video so you can see the patient and the injection.

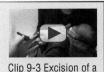

Clip 9-2 Flexor tendon repair in a 10-year-old girl.

- After you inject the local anesthetic, this is what you can tell the patient:

  "I told you all you would feel was one little stick and then no pain.

  I was not lying, was I?"

  They say, "No."

  "I am not lying now. The surgery will not hurt you one little bit now that the magic medicine is in there."

- You can establish a wonderful relationship with most children during WALANT surgery.

- You can avoid all the risks and inconveniences of pediatric sedation and general anesthesia for many cases.

- The same benefits of the patient's seeing active movement in an operation such as flexor tendon repair or a finger fracture holds true for children as for adults.

WALANT HAND SURGERY FOR INFANTS

Clip 9-3 Excision of a fifth finger nubbin in a 4-week-old infant.

- For accessory finger nubbins in a newborn, have the mother start to feed the infant for a minute before gently pinching the skin and inserting the 30-gauge needle under the finger nubbin at the same time. Inject enough 1% lidocaine with 1:100,000 epinephrine with 10% by volume of 8.4% bicarbonate that you can see the tissue swell up under the nubbin. The needle pain momentarily distracts the baby from drinking milk, but he or she usually just carries on feeding quickly because the discomfort is brief and minor.

TIPS AND TRICKS FOR PEDIATRIC WALANT HAND SURGERY

- Start with a 30-gauge needle instead of a 27-gauge needle.

- Have the local anesthetic in your pocket, out of sight and ready to inject, without the child seeing the syringe. Have the child look away before you take the syringe out of your pocket and while you insert the needle.

- Simply pressing firmly on the skin proximal to where you will insert the needle can create sensory input "noise" that decreases the pain felt by the patient. (See Chapter 5 for a list of rules of how to inject local anesthetic with minimal pain.)

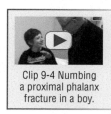

Clip 9-4 Numbing a proximal phalanx fracture in a boy.

NO TOURNIQUET FOR CASES IN WHICH A GENERAL ANESTHETIC IS ADMINISTERED

- The benefits of epinephrine vasoconstriction and painless awakening from the lidocaine also apply when patients are asleep.

- For pediatric repair of a trigger thumb performed under general anesthesia, inject under the skin at the center of the incision until you see the tissues are a little swollen and firm. Usually no more than 1 ml is required in these tiny thumbs.

- For other operations in which children will be having general anesthesia, you can still avoid the tourniquet and let-down bleeding. As soon as the anesthesiologist has the child safely asleep and lets you proceed, inject the lidocaine with epinephrine wherever you will dissect. Then you can go scrub, prep, and drape the patient. By the time you make the first incision, the epinephrine will have started to work.

COMMUNICATION AND INJECTION SKILLS

With a little practice in communication and injection techniques, most hand surgeons can easily provide almost pain-free local anesthesia to children to make their hand surgery experience and that of their parents a safe, pleasurable, and educational one.

CHAPTER 10
FIELD STERILITY FOR SIMPLE CASES MAKES SENSE

Donald H. Lalonde

FIELD STERILITY VERSUS FULL STERILITY

- In this book, *field sterility,* as shown below, means creating a localized sterile field with four towels or a small 40 × 40 cm drape with a hole in it. We only expose and sterilize the part we are operating on or need to see move during the surgery. The surgeon has a mask and sterile gloves, but no sterile gown. Laminar airflow is not required.

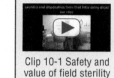

Clip 10-1 Safety and value of field sterility for hand surgery.

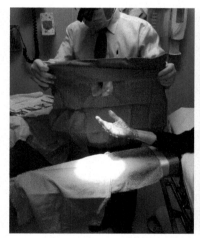 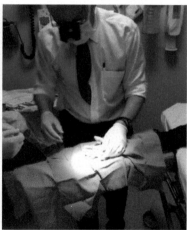

Most carpal tunnel procedures in Canada are performed with field sterility in a minor procedure room outside of the main operating room.

- In this book, *full sterility* means standard operating room full draping with the entire patient covered in sterile drapes, with surgeons and nurses in sterile operating gowns, masks, and gloves.

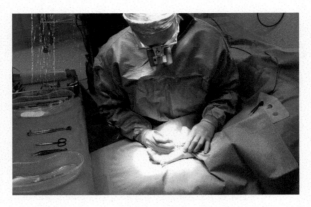

Full sterility for carpal tunnel surgery in the main operating room is half as efficient and four times more expensive.[3]

FULL STERILITY VERSUS FIELD STERILITY FOR MINOR PROCEDURES: WHAT IS THE EVIDENCE?

• Plastic surgeons all over the world have excised small skin cancers and benign lesions with field sterility outside the main operating room for well over 80 years, with no red flags of excessive incidence of infection. The standard of care of Mohs surgery skin cancer excision everywhere in the United States is field sterility outside the main operating room. A recent prospective American cohort study of 20,871 cases of Mohs surgery with field sterility revealed an infection rate of 0.37% with only 78 infections.[1] This infection rate is almost identical to the 1500-case series field sterility carpal tunnel infection rate discussed next.

• What is the evidence for field sterility infection in hand surgery? In a prospective consecutive series of 1504 field sterility carpal tunnel procedures in five North American cities by six surgeons,[2] only six patients developed superficial infections, none of which required incision and drainage; no intravenous antibiotics were given, no reoperation was necessary, and none of the patients required hospital admission. Two infections resolved with suture removal and no antibiotics, and only four patients required oral antibiotics. None of these patients had been given preoperative antibiotics. The infection rate in that 1504-case series was 0.39%, almost identical to the Mohs 20,871-case series described earlier.

• For many years, Canadian hand surgeons have been doing most carpal tunnel and trigger finger operations with field sterility in minor procedure rooms with very few infections.[3] The patient doesn't need to suffer the embarrassment of getting undressed and being transported on a stretcher, although perfectly healthy. There is no monitoring. He or she simply rolls up a sleeve, has the surgery, and then gets up and goes home.

- There is no evidence that outcomes in carpal tunnel surgery are better with full sterility than with field sterility. However, the cost is at least four times as much, the efficiency is half as much, and the garbage production is more than ten times greater.[3]

- Most simple hand trauma operations in Calgary, Saskatoon, Ottawa, Saint John, and other Canadian cities happen with field sterility as well. Those Canadian hand surgeons are repairing tendons and K-wiring most fractures outside the main operating room in clinic procedure rooms Monday through Friday, 8 AM to 5 PM. Calgary has dedicated field sterility clinic trauma rooms on weekend daytime hours as well. Patients may get a better tendon repair at 2 PM than at 2 AM when surgeons and nurses are sleepy.

- Just over a century ago, humans discovered how to safely administer a local anesthetic or induce sedation and general anesthesia to make surgery easier, less painful, and safer. We now know that we don't always need general anesthesia, especially if we are not hurting patients when we inject a local anesthetic. More anesthetic is not always better than less anesthetic. Likewise, more sterility is not necessarily always better than less sterility.

- If we were to follow the premise that more sterility is always better than less sterility, we would all be using "space-suit" sterility measures, as shown below, even for drawing blood or starting an intravenous line. After all, that little plastic intravenous catheter that has contacted bacteria on the skin is placed in a vein with a direct line to the heart! However, we all would agree that we don't need that much sterility for a venipuncture or starting an IV.

- The human and financial cost of an infection after venipuncture or intravenous insertion does not warrant the cost of space-suit sterility, both in terms of human suffering and in dollars. Infections are not common and are usually easily dealt with inexpensively.

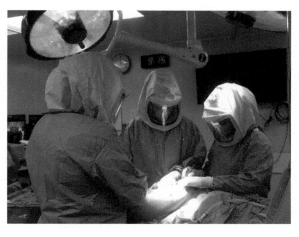

"Space-suit" full operating room sterility is appropriate for insertion of an artificial knee. If a patient's implant becomes infected, the cost is massive both in patient morbidity and in dollars for care. Optimal sterility is worth the investment for that type of operation. In comparison, the cost of an infected carpal tunnel procedure is minimal both in terms of human cost and dollars.

- Where does trigger finger or carpal tunnel surgery fit between drawing blood and knee implant insertion? We need to look at the downside of infection to learn the answer. What are the usual problems associated with infection after carpal tunnel surgery? Not many. Most people respond to suture removal, oral antibiotics, elevation, and immobilization. Very few ever need incision and drainage plus administration of intravenous antibiotics. Most hand surgeons have never seen devastating infection after carpal tunnel surgery because it is so rare. Is it reasonable to spend vast amounts of money for full sterility and millions of tons of medical waste every year to prevent a problem that may not even exist? Probably not.

- We need better evidence, such as the studies cited earlier, to guide the appropriate amount of sterility for which we spend a lot of money. We need to use solid evidence to help us make wise decisions as we fine-tune how much sterility we really need to do each of the various invasive procedures we perform safely. Patients can't afford the cost, surgeons and hospitals can't afford the cost, and the world does not need the garbage produced unnecessarily by the false assumption that more sterility measures are always better.[4]

- When full sterility is required for a procedure such as inserting a permanent PIP joint implant, the wide awake hand operation can be moved to the main operating room or theater with full sterility and laminar airflow.

- The blood supply to the hand is excellent, which is why most hand lacerations sutured in the emergency department do not develop infection, despite the fact that many of those lacerations occurred in severely contaminated hands. Before such lacerations occur, no prepping and draping is done, and no antibiotics are given.

- Now that we no longer need the tourniquet and sedation for hand surgery, field sterility permits us to perform minor hand surgery for carpal tunnel release and minor hand trauma outside the main operating room, which greatly decreases the cost of the surgery[3-6] (see Chapter 11).

WHEN DO WE USE THE MAIN OPERATING ROOM WITH FULL STERILITY FOR HAND SURGERY?

- We perform the vast majority of our hand surgeries in the clinic or office, because using the main operating room is much slower and much more expensive; the only added benefit is absolute sterility. The only time we perform WALANT procedures in the main operating room is when we want that full sterility.

- Examples of cases that we take to the main operating room are plating fractures, thumb basal joint arthroplasty, complex tendon transfers, secondary tendon reconstruction procedures, and similar cases.

- These cases all require either permanent implants or a prolonged operating time in a relatively avascular space, which increases the risk of infection.

References

1. Alam M, Ibrahim O, Nodzenski M, et al. Adverse events associated with Mohs micrographic surgery: multicenter prospective cohort study of 20,821 cases at 23 centers. JAMA Dermatol 149:1378, 2013.
2. Leblanc MR, Lalonde DH, Thoma A, Bell M, Wells N, Allen M, Chang P, Mckee D, Lalonde J. Is main operating room sterility really necessary in carpal tunnel surgery? A multicenter prospective study of minor procedure room field sterility surgery. Hand (N Y) 6:60, 2011.
3. Leblanc MR, Lalonde J, Lalonde DH. A detailed cost and efficiency analysis of performing carpal tunnel surgery in the main operating room versus the ambulatory setting in Canada. Hand (N Y) 2:173, 2007.
4. Sieber D, Lacey A, Fletcher J, Kalliainen L. Cost savings using minimal draping for routine hand procedures. Minn Med 97:49, 2014.
5. Bismil MS, Bismil QM, Harding D, Harris P, Lamyman E, Sansby L. Transition to total one-stop wide-awake hand surgery service-audit: a retrospective review. JRSM Short Rep 3:23, 2012.
6. Chatterjee A, McCarthy JE, Montagne SA, Leong K, Kerrigan CL. A cost, profit, and efficiency analysis of performing carpal tunnel surgery in the operating room versus the clinic setting in the United States. Ann Plast Surg 66:245, 2011.

CHAPTER 11

REVENUES INCREASE AND COSTS DECREASE WITH WALANT

Donald H. Lalonde

THE BOTTOM LINE

- Eliminating the need for a tourniquet (see Chapter 3 and injecting local anesthetic so that it hardly hurts the patient at all (see Chapter 5) removes the two main reasons that patients *need* sedation for most hand operations. Once patients truly understand the added conveniences of WALANT (see Chapter 2), most will no longer *want* sedation for hand surgery, any more than they would want sedation to have a tooth filled at the dentist's.

- Eliminating sedation also means that you can easily perform many hand surgery cases in minor procedure rooms with field sterility in the same way that you remove nevi and small skin cancers (see Chapter 10).

- It is primarily tradition that stands in the way of eliminating the tourniquet, sedation, and the need for main operating room full sterility (see Chapter 12) for hand surgery. Once all concerned have a better understanding that WALANT increases patient safety and convenience while decreasing costs and unnecessary production of garbage, more patients will benefit.

DECREASED COSTS FOR THE PATIENT

- Patients ultimately pay the whole cost of their health care, either directly with cash or indirectly through public taxes or private insurance plan payments. Ultimately, the patient saves all of the costs of sedation or general anesthesia listed here under hospital costs.[1]

- Patients spend less time at the hospital because there is no sedation and because they do not need to undress and be transferred into the main operating room. They roll up their sleeve, have the surgery, then get up and go home right after the operation. Less time at the hospital means less time away from work, lower child care costs, fewer parking fees, and other incidental expenses associated with an overnight or prolonged hospital stay.

- The purpose of most preoperative testing is to increase the safety of sedation rather than to confirm the patient's readiness for surgery. Patients therefore do not incur the cost of time away from work or getting a babysitter while they go for the preoperative assessment or testing required for sedation, because this will not be needed with WALANT.

- Many facilities require patients to have someone stay with them the evening and/or night of sedation. There are no "babysitter" requirements for patients who have wide awake surgery. Patients can go home, look after their children, and resume their normal activities without having someone accompany them to look after them as they recover from sedation.

- Surgeons give patients intraoperative education that may well decrease their risk of complications and reoperation and therefore decrease the costs associated with these events.

- It is possible to see a patient in consultation and operate on him or her the same day, because there is little or no preoperative workup required for pure local anesthesia. This is a significant cost savings for patients who have to travel long distances to the surgeon's facility.[2]

DECREASED COSTS AND INCREASED REVENUE FOR THE SURGEON

- Many surgeons have negotiated with their insurance providers or governments to receive a facility fee or permission to be reimbursed for performing carpal tunnel procedures with WALANT in their offices. Many providers are receptive to the concept of increasing patient safety and convenience while decreasing costs.

- Educating patients while you inject a local anesthetic and operate on them is time you do not need to spend talking to the patient in the office (see Chapter 8).

- Office minor procedure rooms can obtain accreditation by the American Association for Accreditation of Ambulatory Surgery Facilities (AAAASF) in the United States and the Canadian Association for Accreditation of Ambulatory Surgical Facilities (CAAASF) in Canada for procedures using pure local anesthesia (no sedation). Accreditation for an operating room that does not use sedation is much easier and less expensive to obtain than accreditation for a facility that uses sedation or general anesthesia. If you do not use sedation, the costs of equipment and medications related to sedation disappear.

DECREASED COSTS AND INCREASED PROFITABILITY FOR THE HOSPITAL, OPERATING FACILITY, AND THE SURGEON

- If you remove all of the costs of sedation, you eliminate many expenses of traditional hand surgery for the hospital or operating facility. These include the following:
  - Anesthesiologist fees, their allied personnel salaries, and the cost of their medications and equipment
  - In the operating room, salaries for extra nurses who would be required with sedation
  - Salaries for recovery room nurses, because patients simply get up and go home after surgery
  - All of the personnel required to process the sedation (such as patient greeters and test and information processors)
  - Preoperative ECGs, blood tests, chest radiographs, and the salaries of those who perform them
  - Perioperative medical consultation costs required for safe sedation in patients with medical comorbidities
  - Full sterility costs, which are four times higher than for field sterility for carpal tunnel surgery[3]

- Requiring fewer personnel decreases the cost of having the slowest person in the team increase turnover time. A team is only as fast as its slowest member. Each additional team member required for an operation increases the risk that a slower person will get on the team.

- You eliminate the problem of "no beds in recovery/PACU," because there is no "recovery" required from pure local anesthesia with lidocaine and epinephrine.

- One study showed that we could perform twice as many WALANT carpal tunnel procedures in the same time simply by moving the cases outside the main operating room to a minor procedure room with field sterility[2] (see Chapter 10).

- Turnover time is less with field sterility than with full sterility. It takes much less time to set up the cases, walk in the awake patient, and drape him or her.

- There is no need to wash the floor between 5-minute field sterility carpal tunnel procedures or to pay an employee to wash that floor.

- At the hospitals in many cities in Canada (Saint John, Ottawa, Regina, and Calgary), most of the hand trauma surgeries are performed in minor procedure rooms outside of the main operating room with field sterility in daytime hours. Main operating room evening and night time premium costs for doctors, nurses, and other personnel are avoided.

- The risk of litigation decreases, because trauma cases reconstructed during daytime hours are less likely to end up with complications than those operated on at 2 AM because of operator and staff fatigue. In addition, the bond that occurs between the surgeon and the patient with good intraoperative communication and education also decreases the risk of patient discontent and litigation.

- There is less risk of wrong-sided surgery with awake, unsedated patients.

- WALANT trauma surgery in an outpatient clinic or emergency department means that there are no delays waiting for availability of an anesthetist, a scrub team, or a main operating room.

- Intraoperative testing for tendon gapping with active movement after repair has decreased the need for and costs of reoperation for complications such as tendon rupture and tenolysis[2,4] (see Chapter 32).

- Less expensive draping and gowning is required for field sterility (see Chapter 10).

- Disposal of blood-soiled garbage is more expensive than regular garbage disposal. There is less waste disposal of drapes and gowns.

- There is no need for patient gowns, paper footwear, and hats, because patients do not undress for field sterility surgery.

DECREASED COSTS AND INCREASED PROFITABILITY FOR PAYERS: INSURANCE COMPANIES AND GOVERNMENTS

- Eventually, insurance companies and governments will understand that sedation is not necessary for many surgeries of the hand. They will become receptive to the concept of increasing patient safety and convenience while decreasing costs and unnecessary garbage production.[1,5] The payer saves all of the costs previously described.

- Eventually, insurance companies and governments will become aware of evidence-based medicine that supports the concept that much less expensive field sterility is safe for many hand operations. This will decrease their costs by at least 75%[3] (see Chapter 10).

References

1. Bismil MS, Bismil QM, Harding D, Harris P, Lamyman E, Sansby L. Transition to total one-stop wide awake hand surgery service-audit: a retrospective review. JRSM Short Rep 3:23, 2012.

2. Lalonde DH. Wide awake flexor tendon repair and early mobilization in zones 1 and 2. Hand Clin 29:207, 2013.

3. Leblanc MR, Lalonde J, Lalonde DH. A detailed cost and efficiency analysis of performing carpal tunnel surgery in the main operating room versus the ambulatory setting in Canada. Hand (N Y) 2:173, 2007.

4. Higgins A, Lalonde DH, Bell M, McKee D, Lalonde JF. Avoiding flexor tendon repair rupture with intraoperative total active movement examination. Plast Reconstr Surg 126:941, 2010.

5. Chatterjee A, McCarthy JE, Montagne SA, Leong K, Kerrigan CL. A cost, profit, and efficiency analysis of performing carpal tunnel surgery in the operating room versus the clinic setting in the United States. Ann Plast Surg 66:245, 2011.

CHAPTER 12

THE "BUY-IN": ADMINISTRATION, ANESTHESIOLOGY, NURSING, AND PAYERS

Julie E. Adams, Michael W. Neumeister, Robert E. Van Demark, Jr., Carolyn L. Kerrigan, Peter C. Amadio, Donald H. Lalonde

GENERAL STRATEGIES TO MAXIMIZE THE CHANCES OF SUCCESS IN IMPLEMENTING THE CHANGES REQUIRED TO DEVELOP WALANT IN INSTITUTIONS

- Wide awake hand surgery has many benefits for patients, surgeons, facilities, and payers (see Chapter 2). However, making the transition from surgery with sedation requires some adaptation. Developing a strategy to generate institutional buy-in can enhance one's ability to implement this technique into practice.

- Getting buy-in from colleagues, administrators, and payers may require your investing unpaid time to set up meetings with key individuals to show them PowerPoint presentations and appeal to their common sense to do what is best for patients.

- It is best to be prepared with a short but compelling discussion of what you wish to do, why you wish to pursue this route, and what you believe the advantages will be. Feel free to show them the next video clip.

HELP ADMINISTRATORS, NURSES, ANESTHESIOLOGISTS, AND PAYERS UNDERSTAND WALANT

- We have discussed all of the advantages of WALANT versus traditional surgery with sedation and tourniquet in Chapters 2, 8, 9, 10, and 11. Show these chapters and videos to your colleagues, including the references from those chapters, to support the concept.

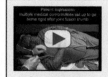

Clip 12-1 Why patients love WALANT.

- Seek out and involve chief stakeholders from the start. It is more effective to arrange one-on-one meetings with videos of PowerPoint presentations with key decision-makers before getting into the committee level.

- Present a succinct but compelling case for why you think it is better for patients, the facility, and other stakeholders.

- Show them the evidence you have for why this is a better way.

- Show them the evidence you have for why it is safe and effective.

- Present it in a respectful way, being certain to listen carefully to objections and concerns.
- Validate their challenges in making change as you address those concerns.
- Be open to discussion and ask the stakeholders what they need from you to make this work. This can go a long way toward garnering goodwill and buy-in.
- It is best to make it a "win-win-win" situation for the stakeholders as well as for you and your patients. Consider the perspective of your facility colleagues and appeal to their needs.
- Be flexible to accept and welcome (or even suggest) small steps toward the desired goal. If leadership will not allow you to start doing wide awake hand surgery in the full extent you desire, but will allow you a trial period or to do so within a more limited basis, that is still a step forward which should be welcomed. As staff and leadership become familiar and comfortable with wide awake surgery, the indications and use can expand.
- Some compelling arguments include that you can improve patient satisfaction ratings, bring more work to the facility, increase the number of patients and cases done in a day, decrease the staff count for many procedures, open up ORs for "bigger" cases, and decrease the amount of wasted materials.
- In some facilities, suggestion of a "pilot study" or "quality improvement project" or "new patient-centered care initiative" to validate what others have done in the literature may help to dissolve resistance.
- Some sample narratives include the following:

  "Would it be OK to try this on a few select patients and see how things go?"

  "Let's do all the monitoring you want initially, and then see if we truly need it."

  "Ok, I understand you don't feel comfortable with this. Can you help me understand why? What parameters would help you feel more comfortable? Why don't we start from that point and see how it goes with a few cases."

Next Steps

- After meeting one-on-one with key leaders, arrange a meeting of the "convinced" to create an action plan to institute the wide awake alternative for at least some of the patients as a starting point. Doing it in small steps may be wiser.
- After you meet with key decision-makers one-on-one, consider creating a WALANT implementation group or committee with all the rest of the stakeholders so they can express their concerns and address them as a group.

Introduction to Nursing Leaders

- Introduce the WALANT concept to nursing leaders and key decision-makers in the perioperative areas with one-on-one PowerPoint presentations and documents. Presentations to the rest of the nursing staff can follow later.

- You can measure improved outcomes:
  - Nausea
  - Vomiting
  - Staff and material costs and waste
  - Patient time in hospital/clinic
  - Patient total cost of surgery
  - Number of times patient has a needle before the surgery
  - Pain of the needle(s) for the patient
  - Did you get to talk to your surgeon the day of surgery?
  - How long were you with the surgeon in a position that you could ask questions?
  - Turnover time
  - Number of patients processed/time
  - Case delay and cancellation statistics

- Discuss cost saving, increased safety with no sedation, increased staff and patient satisfaction, quality improvement, improved efficiency, improved surgeon satisfaction, the overall great experience for the patient and family, and other relevant factors.

Introduction to Anesthesiologists

- Explain to anesthesiologists that WALANT can free them up to provide care for the larger surgeries. Point out to these doctors and to nurses that they personally get no monitoring when they go to the dentist. You are planning to give exactly the same drugs they get at the dentist—only lidocaine and epinephrine within very safe doses.

- Try working with your anesthesiologist to inject only propofol for the 2-minute local anesthetic injection part of the case. The patient could then wake up and participate in movement of reconstructed parts without a tourniquet. You could still educate patients and they would remember if they are not given amnestic agents, which would void their ability and opportunity to receive intraoperative education. In addition, patients would not need nausea-producing opiates.

- Choose quick, uncomplicated procedures to start, such as carpal tunnel or trigger finger surgeries.

- Choose tenolysis, flexor tendon repairs, and EI to EPL tendon transfers early. Operative personnel will thereafter easily understand the advantages of patients being awake, cooperative, and pain free without the tourniquet and sedation. Team members will understand how better outcomes can improve patient care in these operations.

- Choose the first few patients wisely for their good disposition and cooperative demeanor.

- Other good cases to start without sedation are patients with severe medical comorbidities in whom sedation or general anesthesia would be extremely risky.

Early Implementation

- Obtain patient satisfaction surveys to demonstrate patient buy-in early in your implementation process. The literature has good examples of high patient satisfaction.[1-3]

- Have staff satisfaction surveys sent out to nurses to get their input and support.

- The only current option in your facility may be the main operating room with sedation. There may be no place to perform WALANT for hand procedures. Propose a "quality improvement project" that will compare outcomes of carpal tunnel surgeries performed outside of the operating room in a designated procedure room with field sterility and tumescent local anesthesia.

- If there are minor procedure rooms already in existence in which surgeons or dermatologists are removing skin cancers, determine whether you can start by sharing their rooms for carpal tunnel surgery. You can then progress to minor hand trauma.

INSURANCE COMPANIES AND PAYERS

- Find out who the key decision-maker is in the insurance carriers or government payers you deal with.

- Request a meeting with these decision-makers and show them the video clip from this chapter and the documents that explain this new approach, which will increase patient satisfaction and safety while increasing productivity and decreasing costs.

- Negotiate a facility fee or tray fee to perform carpal tunnel surgeries in your minor procedure rooms at the office, surgery center, or hospital. Explain the cost saving (see Chapter 11) when the surgery is taken out of the main operating room and into the office. Surgeons can benefit from collecting the facility fee, and insurance companies can benefit from paying lower facility fees.

- Eventually, insurance companies and governments will understand that sedation and the main operating room are not essential for operations such as carpal tunnel surgery. They will be happy to save the money and increase their client/population safety and satisfaction. It is to their great advantage to negotiate a lower facility fee with you than what they pay the hospital.

PERCEIVED BARRIERS TO ADOPTING WIDE AWAKE HAND SURGERY AND HOW TO ADDRESS THESE ISSUES

GENERAL PERCEIVED BARRIERS

The large number of benefits of WALANT are listed in Chapter 2. Nevertheless, in many practices there will be individuals who perceive barriers to implementation of this technique. We provide suggestions on how to deal with these concerns.

Safe Injection of Epinephrine in the Finger

Many health care workers are still not aware that the old dogma that epinephrine should not be used in the fingers is no longer valid.

Suggestions for Resolution

1. Provide them with Chapter 3 of this book.

2. Provide them with reference papers.[4-8]

3. Demonstrate the reversal of epinephrine vasoconstriction in the finger with phentolamine in your next simple hand operation, such as trigger finger release, as explained and shown in a video in Chapter 3.

4. Show them the clip "History of the rise and fall of the epinephrine danger myth" from Chapter 3.

Safety Concerns for Cardiac Responses to Epinephrine Effects Without Monitoring

Suggestions for Resolution

1. Continue to monitor patients with portable monitors for the first few months of your implementation process. It will eventually become apparent that patients do not need monitoring for lidocaine and epinephrine injection any more than they would at a dentist's office.

2. Make the common-sense argument that monitors have not been used for the millions of lidocaine and epinephrine injections that occur every day without problems in dental offices. Ask the objecting person if he ever had a monitor when he personally had lidocaine with epinephrine at the dentist's.

3. Point out that there are areas in your hospital where doctors inject lidocaine with epinephrine daily without monitors (Mohs surgery clinic, plastic surgery skin cancer and nevus excision, line insertion, and other instances).

4. When patients do have cardiac issues, decrease the concentration of epinephrine to between 1:400,000 to 1:1,000,000 and perform the procedure wide awake in the main operating room with monitors.

5. Give them a copy of Chapter 6, "Dealing With Systemic Adverse Reactions to Lidocaine and Epinephrine."

"My Facility Is Not Set Up So That I Can Inject Patients Before They Come Into the Operating Room"

Ideally, you should inject the local anesthetic at least 20 to 30 minutes before the incision is done to allow optimal epinephrine vasoconstriction.[9] In some facilities, this may present a difficulty in that there is no perceived space available for preoperative blocking.

Suggestions for Resolution

1. Although 20 to 30 minutes is ideal, you can begin a procedure sooner than that if necessary. You will need to tolerate initial temporary bleeding, which is only mildly annoying.

2. You can inject patients on stretchers in any preoperative holding area or in the recovery room.

3. You can inject patients as soon as they arrive in the operating room before you scrub and prepare and drape the patient.

4. Dr. Robert Van Demark, Jr., of Sanford USD Medical Center, Sioux Falls, South Dakota, recently persuaded his hospital to renovate a location for wide awake hand surgery. See Dr. Van Demark's comments in this chapter for details.

"My Facility Requires a Witnessed Preinjection Time Out or Pause: This May Be Difficult If I Inject Local Anesthetic Outside the Operating Room"

Suggestions for Resolution

1. Start by performing the injections in the holding area or recovery room with a nurse there as a witness. They will probably eventually come around to seeing that this may not be necessary in an awake patient.

2. Point out that we developed the concept of time out in operating rooms mostly to protect patients from the risks of sedative medication. Patients cannot protect themselves while in a sedated state. When a patient is totally awake, he or she can and likely would answer the questions of health care providers. Although still possible, wrong-sided operations are much less likely.

3. Point out that there are places in your hospital outside the operating room where doctors inject local anesthetics in unsedated patients without time outs.

PATIENT-PERCEIVED BARRIERS

It will be essential to change the culture of patients' expectations: perhaps a family member or friend had sedation for the same surgery and they feel they need sedation.

Most Patient Concerns Arise From Fear of the Unknown

Suggestions for Resolution

A calm, confident attitude with soft-spoken, straightforward explanations of the truth about how simple WALANT hand surgery can be is very reassuring for patients. Explain that the safest sedation is no sedation. Use the strategies discussed in Chapter 7 and point out all the benefits of being awake from Chapter 2.

Fear of Pain

Suggestions for Resolution

1. Explain to patients that advances in local anesthesia make it possible that smaller local anesthetic needles (27- or 30-gauge) hurt less than the larger intravenous cannula needles commonly used for sedation (20-gauge).

2. Tell them that the only pain they will likely feel is one little stick from a tiny needle—and then deliver on that promise as outlined in Chapter 5. Score yourself each time you inject local anesthetic so you can consistently deliver minimally painful injections.

Fear of Knowing What the Surgeon Is Doing, Hearing Noises and Conversations

Suggestions for Resolution

Explain to patients that they can chose to know or not know what the surgeon is doing, as they wish. If they would like to be totally "out of the know," they can bring in music with headphones and ignore the whole event. If they change their mind and would like a "play-by-play" of the surgery, this can easily be accommodated by experienced wide awake surgeons. Many patients do like to see parts of their surgery.

NURSE-PERCEIVED BARRIERS

It will be necessary to change the culture of nurses: most of their concerns are a result of the fact that they have never tried the wide awake approach. Most of the perceived issues go away quickly after even a short exposure to the technique.

Most Nursing Concerns Come From Fear of the Unknown

Suggestions for Resolution

1. As a first step, meet one-on-one with key administrative nurses, as outlined earlier in this chapter.

2. Have the nurses who seem more receptive to the WALANT concept be the first to try a few cases.

Claustrophobia From the Drapes

Suggestions for Resolution

Explain to the nurses that draping is there to protect the patients and decrease the potential of infection, not to drive patients crazy or unnerve them. Draping that leaves the head free of drapes can easily accommodate the concerns of such patients and maintain an ample sterile field.[10]

What Happens If the Patient Feels Pain?

Suggestions for Resolution

The surgeon can always inject more local anesthetic and the pain will go away. If the surgeon follows the simple guidelines of tumescent local anesthetic administration (see Chapter 4) and minimal pain injection of local anesthetic (see Chapter 5), this should be as infrequent as patients waking up during general anesthesia. The only reasons patients may feel pain during the surgery are that an insufficient volume of anesthetic solution was injected or insufficient time was allowed for the local anesthetic to take effect. Just as airline pilots always make sure they have enough fuel to land at an alternate airport, surgeons or anesthesiologists giving the local anesthetic should always be prepared to be able to inject more local anesthetic volume while staying within the safe dosage limit.

If the Surgery Is More Difficult Than Anticipated, How Do They Calm the Patient? Are the Nurses Responsible for Conversing With the Patient?

Suggestions for Resolution

Nurses and surgeons both become responsible for creating a calm, relaxed environment for the patient. Nurses will now communicate directly with the patient for many things that they used to communicate with the anesthesiologist and the surgeon. In practice, the patient is easily calmed if the surgeon and the nurse are relaxed with a matter-of-fact attitude. Surgeons and nurses who cannot remain calm and confident should likely not embark on surgery with a wide awake patient. The very worst case scenario that may occur is that the surgeon might not be able to finish a case unless he gets a general anesthetic for his patient. This would only occur with poor patient selection and has never occurred in our practices. If it did occur, we would simply close the skin and reschedule the patient for a safe, no-rush procedure with a general anesthetic.

Will Fewer Nurses Be Needed?

Suggestions for Resolution

We may need fewer nurses with no sedation procedures, because many of the problems that nurses solve are sedation- and general anesthesia–induced issues. The surgical roles of the nurses do not change.

Are Nurses Liable If a Medical Emergency Happens?

Suggestions for Resolution

Nurses are no more liable in medical emergencies in wide awake patients than they are for medical emergencies with patients in the holding area or in the rest of the hospital.

SURGEON-PERCEIVED BARRIERS

Changing the culture of surgeons: Most of the concerns of surgeons are a result of the fact that they have never tried the wide awake approach. Most of the perceived issues go away quickly after even a short exposure to the technique.

"I Cannot Work at My Facility Unless I Have an Anesthesiologist in the Room"

Suggestions for Resolution

Ask your anesthesia provider to limit the injection to propofol for the 2 minutes required for you to inject the lidocaine and epinephrine. As soon as you have injected the local anesthetic, the anesthesiologist can wake the patient. Avoiding all amnestics and opiates will allow you to teach patients during the injection and the procedure and have them remember your advice. They will not have nausea. They will also be able to cooperate and show you movement of reconstructed structures without the motor block. Alternatively, your anesthesiologist may change his or her role to that of a consultant who is not necessarily present for your whole case.

"I Don't Get Paid the Same If I Use WALANT"

Suggestions for Resolution

Set up meetings with your local insurance company executives or government payers, as other surgeons have. Make the business case about how the use of pure local anesthetic will cost them much less in the end. Negotiate with them to give you a facility fee to do the carpal tunnels in your office that would cost them less than the facility fee at a hospital but make it worth your efforts. (See Dr. Kerrigan's comments in this chapter.)

Surgeons Will Now Be Forced to Talk to the Patient During Surgery

Suggestions for Resolution

You can keep conversation to a minimum, but it is true that the wide awake approach does pressure surgeons to talk to patients during surgery. If you are the type of surgeon who does not like this type of interaction, perhaps WALANT is not for you. However, this can be an excellent intraoperative opportunity for patient teaching to decrease the risk of unnecessary postoperative complications (see Chapter 8).

Patients Hear Conversations in the Operating Room

Suggestions for Resolution

Patients can hear what the operating room staff are saying. You must take greater care in how you speak. See Chapter 8 for suggestions about things to say and not to say in the operating room when patients are listening.

Difficult Surgeries Are More Transparent to the Patients

Suggestions for Resolution

Transparency about the difficulty of surgery is not necessarily a bad thing. When patients see a surgeon struggle to perform a difficult case, they gain an appreciation for the delicate nature of the problem. They understand more readily why it may be difficult to get a perfect result. This has often worked in our favor, because patients become more realistic in their expectations and accepting of the limitations of surgery.

The Patient Knows When Residents or Students Are Participating in Their Surgery

Suggestions for Resolution

We have found that many patients gain a great respect for their good fortune in having a master responsible for their surgery when they see a surgeon teaching a resident to do part of a case. If the surgeon has a calm, reassuring manner, this can be a very positive experience for the patient. On the other hand, if a surgeon is rough and aggressive in his teaching technique, the patient may be better off asleep.

1. Start by teaching the resident or medical student how to inject the local anesthetic in a minimally painful way, as shown in Chapter 5. The patient will then be quite amazed at how little pain he or she felt during local anesthesia injection by the learner and will likely become

much more willing to have the trainee do parts or all of the case under the surgeon's supervision.

2. For things to say and do while teaching residents during WALANT, see Chapter 8.

3. It is true that the patient will be much more aware of who did which parts of the surgery, especially if the surgeon is not there for part of the operation. This increased transparency and truth-revealing to patients may be too much for the surgeon to bear, in which case the surgeon may prefer to have the patient asleep.

The Patient Is Aware of Inefficiencies in the Operating Room Such as Delays, Dropped Instruments, and Lack of Needed Equipment

Suggestions for Resolution

Unforeseen things do occur, and personnel enter and leave the operating room. This is just part of the normal workaday life of a surgical team. When things go slightly awry, we can convey a sense of matter-of-fact calm that will reassure the patient with our attitude and our reaction to adversity. In this way patients will witness us at our best behavior, not at our worst behavior.

ANESTHESIOLOGIST-PERCEIVED BARRIERS

Changing the culture of anesthesiologists: Most of the concerns of anesthesiologists are a result of the fact that they have never tried the wide awake approach. Most of the perceived issues go away quickly after even a short exposure to the technique.

"How Do I Fit Into This?"

Suggestions for Resolution

1. If anesthesiologists only give propofol for the local anesthetic injection part and then wake the patient up, the patient feels no local anesthetic injection pain and retains the benefits of the awake patient getting intraoperative education and cooperation, with minimal nausea.

2. Alternatively, anesthesiologists who are interested in developing skills in the injection of tumescent local anesthetic without sedation are more than welcome to start using the technique. This would free up surgeon time. Anesthesiologists could be injecting local anesthetic outside the procedure room while the surgeon operates on patients in the procedure room. Anesthesiologists and surgeons may want to convince payers that they should cover this service if they do not already.

3. An anesthesiologist may change his or her role to that of a consultant who is not necessarily present for your whole case.

"What If They Call Me Into a Room Where WALANT Surgery Is Being Performed to Look After a Medical Problem in a Patient I Have Never Met Before?"

Suggestions for Resolution

This would be the same as if a patient they had not met had a medical problem in the preoperative holding area. None of the medical issues arises from sedation. Hence the anesthesiologist may not necessarily need to become involved. The surgeon can transfer the patient to other doctors to look after the medical problem.

"My Income May Decline"

Suggestions for Resolution

It is true that anesthesiologists' income may decline if they do not adapt to sedation-free tumescent local anesthesia. However, this is not a good reason to avoid WALANT surgery if it is better overall for patient care.

Pain Management May Be Out of Control

Suggestions for Resolution

In reality, this problem does not occur in practice. The surgeon can always provide more local anesthetic if it is required. In addition, surgeons are very capable of managing pain control with systemic medication. In fact, WALANT eliminates intraoperative systemic pain medications and their adverse effects.

"Sedation Is Better for Patients Than Pure Local Anesthesia"

Suggestions for Resolution

It is true that sedation with an anesthesiologist is safer than sedation without an anesthesiologist. However, it is not true that sedation is safer than no sedation. In fact, it is quite the opposite. All anesthesiologists will agree that less sedation is safer than more sedation. The logical conclusion is that the safest sedation is no sedation. Dental offices have used only lidocaine with epinephrine very safely for over 60 years without monitoring. Wrong-sided surgery is much less likely to occur in unsedated patients than in those who are asleep or heavily sedated. All anesthesiologists struggle with the problem of nausea and vomiting. The wide awake sedation-free approach eliminates the nausea and vomiting issue.[1]

What Happens If the Patient Loses an Airway?

Suggestions for Resolution

Patients who are receiving pure local anesthetic with lidocaine and epinephrine in the hand will not lose an airway. Even when dentists are actually obstructing the airway with dental procedures in their offices, the loss of an airway in that unmonitored setting is extremely rare, especially if there is no sedation.

PERCEIVED BARRIERS FROM THE CULTURE OF "SURGERY NEEDS SEDATION"

"We've Always Done It This Way: Operating Rooms Need a Surgeon and an Anesthesiologist" and "My Facility Won't Let Me Into an Operating Room Without an Anesthesiologist"

Suggestions for Resolution

Many hospital operating rooms have dedicated "local anesthesia" rooms where surgeons operate safely without any anesthesiology personnel. Other hospitals have still not done it this way. Point out to concerned personnel that dentists work under pure local anesthesia without an anesthesiologist. Local anesthesia without monitoring occurs in many other parts of the hospital for skin cancer excision, minor procedures in the emergency department, and procedures such as bone marrow aspiration.

"Sedation Controls Patients for Their Own Protection"

Suggestions for Resolution

Those of us who have been practicing wide awake surgery understand that most patients adapt very well to pure local anesthesia. Most do not require "protection" from the reality of surgery.

"Sedation Improves Patient Satisfaction"

Suggestions for Resolution

There is no evidence that patients who receive sedation are more satisfied than those who do not. In fact, there is level III evidence that patients who have had wide awake carpal tunnel surgery are just as satisfied as those who received sedation. However, those who had wide awake surgery had less preoperative testing, less narcotic use, less nausea and vomiting, and less time at the hospital.

What About Patient Safety Checklists?

Suggestions for Resolution

We can still perform the safety checklist with an awake patient. In fact, the patient becomes part of the checklist process. We created patient safety checks because operating room staff made mistakes such as wrong-sided surgery, giving patients medications that they were allergic to, and other errors. Most of these issues actually arise because we have sedated patients who cannot speak for themselves and protect themselves. If the only medications that are given are lidocaine and epinephrine with no sedation, most of these operating room errors go away.

OBSERVATIONS FROM SURGEONS WHO PRACTICE WIDE AWAKE HAND SURGERY

Dr. Carolyn L. Kerrigan, Dartmouth-Hitchcock Medical Center, Lebanon, New Hampshire

- Patients are generally not concerned, because I feel comfortable and confident with the approach, as does the team of clinic nurses who support me. We take a very matter-of-fact approach to explaining what will happen; I just calmly explain the "usual" process. Since I feel confident, it is rarely a problem. If they raise the question about sedation, I engage them in a conversation comparing it to WALANT. We discuss having to be fasting, needing to have an IV line started, needing a driver, needing to stop certain medications, needing to get completely undressed, and needing to be wheeled on a stretcher. All these things may make a patient feel more vulnerable and less in control. A small number of patients express anxiety and a desire to take a mild anxiolytic prior to the procedure, and I support them in this.

HOW I GOT OVER OBSTACLES WITH ADMINISTRATION

I had been doing hand procedures under local, with a tourniquet, and with a single nurse in the operating room in a Canadian setting before moving to New Hampshire. I learned and experienced that with a local anesthetic, one nurse, and a lean set of instruments, I could do many different types of hand procedures. When I moved to Dartmouth 18 years ago, it was natural to do carpal tunnel and trigger fingers in the clinic setting. One of the other surgeons was already doing this—the big change for the nurses and administration was that I wanted to do endoscopic procedures outside the main operating room. Initially, they told me that this would be impossible. It took some convincing, borrowing equipment from the operating room, and developing a business case for return on investment until the administrators understood the advantage to patients and the financial bottom line.

HOW I GOT OVER STUMBLING BLOCKS WITH NURSES

Patience and persistence. Ask them to try it once. Make sure that you start with a nurse who has OR experience. Give them training to the competency. For a nurse who has never been in an operating room, it is intimidating to set up a sterile field, open a tray of surgical instruments and assist at surgery. Find an early adopter and you will gradually win over their peers when they see how easy and uncomplicated it is for patients compared to what they have had to do before.

HOW I GET PAID

I work in an academic medical center. Our clinic is physically attached to the inpatient hospital. There is a revenue management group that oversees all the billing and coding for the organization. They track a provider's productivity based on RVUs (relative value units). Charges, payments, payer mix, technical fees are also considered during budget time and throughout the year. The treatment rooms in our clinic are designated as a "provider-based entity." This is an organizational classification, granted through the Centers for Medicare and Medicaid Services (CMS), which identifies services rendered in specifically designated locations as "hospital based." This allows for a system of reimbursement that supports maximization of Part B reimbursement and Part A reimbursement of the technical components of the charge. Our organization can thus bill CMS and commercial payers for both professional and technical fees. There is a specific process to go through to get this designation, and you will need to work with your hospital administrator (at our hospital this was the Senior Manager of Reimbursement) to know if it is possible and to make it happen.*

Dr. Peter C. Amadio, Mayo Clinic, Rochester, Minnesota

- WALANT surgery is resource friendly, because "wide awake" means no or less need for sedating medications that prolong stays in ambulatory care facilities and increase the utilization of nursing staff

- Academic centers can be good places to introduce wide awake techniques, because they are under greater competition for resources but manage more complex cases. Managing patients with less complex resources is thus critically important.

- Local anesthesia means no or much less intense involvement of anesthesiologists and their teams, operating room staff, and recovery room staff.

- Not using a tourniquet saves on both resources and time, since hemostasis is a part of the anesthetic technique rather than being achieved with cautery, ligatures, or other methods. This reduces operative time, and possibly even postoperative hematoma.

- No tourniquet also means no tourniquet pain, no risk of tourniquet palsy, and no risk of skin problems under the tourniquet.

- I frequently use the LANT (local anesthesia no tourniquet) part of WALANT even when patients are asleep. As soon as the patient is anesthetized, we inject the lidocaine and epinephrine where we will dissect. The epinephrine provides hemostasis so there is no let-down bleeding from the tourniquet if we inflate it. The local anesthesia means that less nausea-producing medication from the anesthesiologist is required.

---

*You can find guidance at *https://www.cms.gov/Regulations-and-Guidance/Guidance/Transmittals/downloads/a03030.pdf*.

- Injecting local anesthesia in the holding area both allows more time for the hemostatic effect of the epinephrine to work and means you do not waste time and money in the operating room inducing anesthesia.

- Surgeons need to set aside less time for postoperative teaching when patients observe and participate in their surgery.

- There is little high-level evidence published to date to document better outcomes or patient satisfaction with WALANT, compared with more traditional alternatives. Nevertheless, in my own practice, I have developed certain indications where I believe that WALANT, or variants of it, add value.

- My top indications for WALANT are in such cases as tendon repair, tendon transfer, tendon graft, and tenolysis. In these cases with long tourniquet times, we need patient cooperation. Beyond 10 or 15 minutes, tourniquet pain and paralysis limit the usefulness of a local anesthesia approach. WALANT finesses this by eliminating the tourniquet altogether and allows the patient to remain comfortable, awake, and with full motor control of the hand. This motor control is very important to check tension, pull-through, and integrity of tendon repairs under voluntary load. It is useful to verify complete lysis of adhesions, some of which may be well proximal or distal to the initial zone of injury.

- From a patient education perspective, the patient knows everything that is going on, especially if he or she watches (which I always encourage). A better-informed patient is a happier patient and a better partner in postoperative recovery.

- Most important, patient cooperation is the key to setting tension and checking motion after any kind of tendon surgery and in confirming active motion after contracture releases.

- I have found WALANT to be helpful in having the patient help me set the correct angle for various osteotomies, especially derotational osteotomies of the fingers.

- I have more recently used WALANT when doing trapezium excisions, to assess stability with active pinch after excision and capsular closure, and before performing any ligament reconstruction or other stabilization procedure. I believe that this helps me better "personalize" the procedure to each patient, rather than routinely either not doing a reconstruction, as much of the literature recommends, or routinely doing so, as many continue to do in practice.

- My second main indication for WALANT is for cases in which intraoperative patient teaching could be helpful in managing the postoperative course. In fact, this may actually be almost every case one does, since even for shorter cases such as carpal tunnel or trigger finger, pointing out tendons, nerves, what we do, why, and how we do it intraoperatively affects postoperative activity. This can have a major impact on patient understanding, cooperation, and satisfaction.

- One limit is the length of the case. Few patients can tolerate many hours of lying still on the operating table when fully awake, even if their hand does not hurt. Having said that, we do encourage patients to change their position if they are uncomfortable on the table. We have good access to the hand whether they are on their back or on their side.

- One major indication for WALANT is for cases in which a tourniquet is contraindicated but a bloodless field would be helpful. This would include patients with lymphedema or dialysis access. Another would be upper limb posttraumatic revascularization surgery with the need for additional reconstruction. This avoids any risk that tourniquet may pose to the integrity of the vascular reconstruction.

- Another major indication for WALANT is for a patient receiving anticoagulants. The epinephrine in the anesthetic adds to the reliability of hemostasis in these cases. By the time the epinephrine effect is gone in 4 to 6 hours, even a patient with reduced thrombogenesis will have formed a clot.

- In my own experience with WALANT over the past 5 years in patients aged 12 to 92, I have not had any WALANT-related complications and have yet to have recourse to phentolamine to reverse epinephrine vasoconstriction. Hemostasis has not been a problem.

- I have been especially pleased that my patients seem to enjoy the experience. The following types of comments are common.

    "Thanks, doctor. I really enjoyed the surgery!"

    "Could I have a DVD of the operation?" Usually this is as a memento, but again not infrequently the reason is given as "I want to explain it to my family," which makes me especially happy, because it shows that the patient understands what has just transpired well enough to communicate it to others.

    "People definitely need to put this on their 'bucket list.' It was great!"

- In summary, I have found WALANT to be very useful. The technique allows me to better personalize the care I provide to each patient, engages the patients in their care, and has low morbidity.

Dr. Robert E. Van Demark, Jr., Sanford School of Medicine, The University of South Dakota, Sioux Falls, South Dakota

- I am an orthopedic surgeon employed by a large Midwestern health system. In my practice, there are 13 orthopedists, 2 podiatrists, 2 primary care sports medicine physicians and 19 midlevel providers. Our hospital has 29 operating rooms, with an additional 6 operating rooms devoted to orthopedics.

- Because of the rapid growth of our group, we began to have operating room access problems in 2013. At the same time, we started using WALANT for some of our hand cases. It became apparent that we could move some of those cases out of the hospital setting and do them in our office with WALANT. We could build a procedure room in our office at a fraction of the cost of a new operating room in the hospital ($15,000 versus $5 million). The challenge was to convince all of the stakeholders that building a procedure room in the hospital would be a win-win-win for everyone.

- When we approached hospital leadership, they were reluctant to proceed with plans for a minor procedure room. We needed to address four issues:

    1. What is WALANT surgery?
    2. Is WALANT surgery safe for patients?
    3. Will patients be satisfied with WALANT surgery?
    4. Did this make financial sense for the System?

What Is WALANT Surgery?

Initially there was some confusion concerning wide awake anesthesia. The hospital administration thought we were planning to move a hospital operating room to a procedure room. We needed to educate the administration on what constitutes WALANT surgery. The concept of "minor procedure room field sterility surgery" is new to many outside the spheres of Mohs surgery and plastic surgery in the United States, but Canadian hand surgeons have used it extensively for a long time.[10] Field sterility includes the following components:

- Extremity preparation with iodine or chlorhexidine
- A single drape
    - Minor instrument tray
    - Sterile masks and gloves with no gowns
    - No prophylactic antibiotics
    - Local anesthesia only

Is WALANT Surgery Safe for Patients?

Multiple studies have looked at the safety of doing wide awake hand surgery in the outpatient setting. In a large multicenter study of 1504 carpal tunnel procedures from Canada, the superficial infection rate was 0.4% and the deep infection rate was 0.0%. These findings are similar to the results of other reported series.[11,12]

Will Patients Be Satisfied With WALANT Surgery?

Multiple studies have demonstrated high patient satisfaction.[1-3] A two-center study compared the patient's perspective of wide awake anesthesia and local anesthesia with sedation. In comparing the two groups, sedated patients spent more time in the hospital, required more preoperative testing, and reported greater nausea and vomiting postoperatively. The majority of patients in both groups (93%) liked the anesthesia they had received and would choose it again.[1]

A British study examined the patient experience reviewed in 100 consecutive patients undergoing wide awake hand surgery. Most (91%) felt that the procedure was less painful or comparable to what they would experience from a dental visit; 86% would prefer to have wide awake anesthesia if they needed hand surgery again; and 90% would recommend WALANT to a friend.[2]

Does This Make Financial Sense for the System?
Data have been published on the significant financial savings of using a procedure room instead of a hospital operating room. Costs associated with an anesthesiologist, preoperative testing, IV sedation, intraoperative monitoring, and recovery room personnel go away with the use of local anesthetic.[13-15]

ADDITIONAL EVIDENCE

• In addition to the cost savings, WALANT surgery is more efficient. In one Canadian study, they performed twice as many carpal tunnel releases at one quarter the cost by doing surgery in a minor procedure room instead of the main hospital operating room.[14] An American study showed similar findings.[13] A study from the U.K. reviewed 1000 patients treated with wide awake anesthesia for hand surgery and showed a savings of £750,000 ($1,160,000) for the National Health Service. Over a 10-year period, there was a total savings of £2 million.[16]

• Under the current reimbursement model, some hospitals have little interest in adopting wide awake anesthesia. All of this is about to change. With the passage of the Accountable Care Act (ACA) in 2010, there will be a paradigm shift in reimbursement. There will be a shift from volume to value to control health care costs and to improve the quality (outcomes) of care.[17,18] One of the goals of the ACA is to "control costs by regulating health care delivery and reimbursement."[17] As part of the ACA, Accountable Care Organizations (ACOs) will play a major role in this transition. An ACO is a network of health care providers that provides care to a defined group of patients. To achieve ACO designation, the following guidelines need to be met[17]:
  – "Express willingness to be accountable for quality, cost, and overall care of Medicare beneficiaries for minimum of three years"
  – "Minimum of 5000 Medicare beneficiaries with a strong core of primary care physicians"
  – "Legal structure to receive and allocate payments"
  – "Report on quality, cost, care-coordination measures, and meet patient-centeredness criteria"

• ACOs will be financially responsible for this group of patients. ACOs may be at risk for losing money if costs are higher than expected. In addition, Medicare and insurers will offer financial rewards for saving money and meeting quality guidelines.[17] Payment to ACOs will be an amount equal to a percentage of money saved through cost efficiency.[17]

• When faced with this new economic reality of ACOs and bundled payments, hospitals and health care systems will be interested in adopting new delivery systems that can be cost-effective while providing quality care with high patient satisfaction.

RESOLUTION

- We began by marketing this option to Workers Compensation carriers for local hand cases (as suggested by our vice-president). We are confident that our community will receive this well.

- Regardless of the final form and function of the ACA, we feel prepared for the future. A dedicated procedure room for WALANT will give our patients safe, quality care with excellent outcomes and high patient satisfaction.

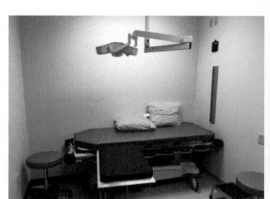
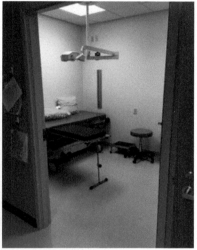
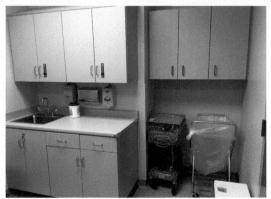

After lengthy discussions, our administration agreed to renovate a hospital room into our new WALANT procedure room. They put two walls in a preexisting large cast room to make it work, and it is functioning well for us at very little cost.

References

1. Davison PG, Cobb T, Lalonde DH. The patient's perspective on carpal tunnel surgery related to the type of anesthesia: a prospective cohort study. Hand (N Y) 8:47, 2013.
2. Teo I, Lam W, Muthayya P, Steele K, Alexander S, Miller G. Patients' perspective of wide-awake hand surgery—100 consecutive cases. J Hand Surg Eur 38:992, 2013.
3. Koegst WH, Wölfle O, Thoele K, Sauerbier M. [The "wide awake approach" in hand surgery: a comfortable anaesthesia method without a tourniquet] Handchir Mikrochir Plast Chir 43:175, 2011.
4. Thomson CJ, Lalonde DH, Denkler KA, Feicht AJ. A critical look at the evidence for and against elective epinephrine use in the finger. Plast Reconstr Surg 119:260, 2007.
5. Lalonde DH, Bell M, Benoit P, Sparkes G, Denkler K, Chang P. A multicenter prospective study of 3,110 consecutive cases of elective epinephrine use in the fingers and hand: the Dalhousie Project clinical phase. J Hand Surg Am 30:1061, 2005.
6. Fitzcharles-Bowe C, Denkler K, Lalonde D. Finger injection with high-dose (1:1,000) epinephrine: does it cause finger necrosis and should it be treated? Hand (N Y) 2:5, 2007.
7. Nodwell T, Lalonde DH. How long does it take phentolamine to reverse adrenaline-induced vasoconstriction in the finger and hand? A prospective randomized blinded study: the Dalhousie project experimental phase. Can J Plast Surg 11:187, 2003.
8. Chowdhry S, Seidenstricker L, Cooney DS, Hazani R, Wilhelmi BJ. Do not use epinephrine in digital blocks: Myth or truth? Part II. A retrospective review of 1111 cases. Plast Reconstr Surg 126:2031, 2010.
9. McKee DE, Lalonde DH, Thoma A, Glennie DL, Hayward JE. Optimal time delay between epinephrine injection and incision to minimize bleeding. Plast Reconstr Surg 131:811, 2013.
10. Leblanc MR, Lalonde DH, Thoma A, Bell M, Wells N, Allen M, Chang P, Mckee D, Lalonde J. Is main operating room sterility really necessary in carpal tunnel surgery? A multi-center prospective study of minor procedure room field sterility surgery. Hand (N Y) 6:60 2011.
11. Hanssen AD, Amadio PC, DeSilva SP, Ilstrup DM. Deep postoperative wound infection after carpal tunnel release. J Hand Surg Am 14:869, 1989.
12. Harness NG, Inacio MC, Pfeil FF, Paxton LW. Rate of infection after carpal tunnel release surgery and effect of antibiotic prophylaxis. J Hand Surg Am 35:189, 2010.
13. Chatterjee A, McCarthy JE, Montagne SA, Leong K, Kerrigan CL. A cost, profit, and efficiency analysis of performing carpal tunnel surgery in the operating room versus the clinic setting in the United States. Ann Plast Surg 66:245, 2011.
14. Leblanc MR, Lalonde J, Lalonde DH. A detailed cost and efficiency analysis of performing carpal tunnel surgery in the main operating room versus the ambulatory setting in Canada. Hand (N Y) 2:173, 2007.
15. Lalonde D, Martin A. Tumescent local anesthesia for hand surgery: improved results, cost effectiveness, and wide-awake patient satisfaction. Arch Plast Surg 41:312, 2014.
16. Bismil MS, Bismil QM, Harding D, Harris P, Lamyman E, Sansby L. Transition to total one-stop wide-awake hand surgery service-audit: a retrospective review. JRSM Short Rep 3:23, 2012.
17. Adkinson JM, Chung KC. The Patient Protection and Affordable Care Act: a primer for hand surgeons. Hand Clin 30:345, 2014.
18. Mathews A. Can accountable-care organizations improve health care while reducing costs? Wall Street Journal, Jan 23, 2012.

CHAPTER 13

PERFORMING YOUR FIRST CASES WITH WALANT

Andrew W. Gurman, Robert E. Van Demark, Jr., Günter Germann, Jason Wong, Donald H. Lalonde

SUGGESTIONS ON GETTING STARTED

Andrew W. Gurman

There are a number of wonderful descriptions in this book about WALANT and its use in some very complex surgical procedures. Chapter 1 offers an atlas with clear descriptions of exactly where to place injections of local anesthetic, how much to inject, and the correct formulation of injectate. For someone who has not used WALANT techniques, getting started can seem formidable. Here are some lessons I learned that I hope are helpful.

- Choose your first cases carefully. Start small: trigger fingers, carpal tunnel releases, first dorsal compartments, simple masses, and skin lesions. Even if you never use WALANT for larger cases, this will still encompass a significant percentage of your schedule.

- Choose your first patients carefully. Let them know what you are planning, and tell them that they are the first on whom you are using the technique. You have used local anesthesia before, so it's OK to tell them that, and explain that the addition of epinephrine means that you may not have to use a tourniquet.

- Put a tourniquet on the arm for your first few cases. You won't use it, but it's comforting to have it in place until you see for yourself how well this works. As a corollary, you can place the tourniquet for more complex surgeries and only inflate it for very brief periods when needed.

- I still use a Penrose drain as a digital tourniquet for digital mucous cysts and nail bed cases. Patients do not feel it with a good digital block. (See Chapters 1, 4, and 5.)

- Stay in your comfort zone. It takes a while to get comfortable with WALANT for some cases. If you have any doubts about a particular case, have the appropriate anesthesia personnel available in case you need to convert to general anesthesia.

THE USE OF **WALANT** TECHNIQUES IN CONJUNCTION WITH GENERAL ANESTHESIA

- I still use general anesthesia for most large cases. However, injection of lidocaine and epinephrine improves results in these cases as well. I would like to acknowledge the work of David L. Nelson, MD, in Marin County, California on postoperative pain management for providing the basis of this practice. (See *http:www.DavidLNelson.MD.*)

- We all witness observable responses to painful stimuli, such as pulse rate increases, blood pressure elevation, and limb withdrawal in patients under general anesthesia. These hard-wired events occur even when sedation alters consciousness. WALANT techniques stop pain impulses from the tourniquet and nerve stimulation. The brain never experiences the "attack" of surgery. Patients need fewer drugs during the operation. This makes waking up and recovery time faster and much easier. Patients need less postoperative opioids (which may induce nausea), particularly if these are combined with a perioperative regimen of acetaminophen and nonsteroidal antiinflammatory agents.

- I inject local anesthetic in the holding area, just as for WALANT cases, or after induction of general anesthesia, before prepping and draping the patient. The advantage of injection in the holding area is that the tumescent fluid spreads in the tissues, and hemostasis improves because the epinephrine has longer to induce vasoconstriction. However, some patients will not tolerate the injections while conscious, or the condition of the limb may require induction of anesthesia before it is unwrapped or manipulated.

- Although the use of bupivacaine is not a part of WALANT technique for smaller cases, I inject 0.5% bupivacaine with epinephrine in the deep layers as well as in the skin while closing larger cases, which helps with postoperative pain control. (See Chapter 6 for more information on longer-lasting local anesthetics.)

TAKING THE FIRST STEP

Robert E. Van Demark, Jr.

Perhaps the biggest obstacle to starting WALANT surgery is taking the first step. If you started practice before 2005, you probably weren't exposed to the WALANT concept in your training. Like me, you probably have done most of your ambulatory surgery cases with a combination of intravenous regional anesthesia, local with sedation, and/or general anesthesia. Usually this has worked well, except for the patients who had tourniquet pain and narcotic hangovers with nausea and vomiting. That is no longer the case when you perform the surgery with local injection only of 1% lidocaine with 1:100,000 epinephrine.

- Patients can have breakfast, take their medications, and drive to and from the hospital or surgery center for their procedure. One of my patients, an 85-year-old with diabetes, drove to the hospital, underwent a carpal tunnel release with WALANT, and drove himself home. (However, see Chapter 7 for the potential legal problems to be addressed with patients using this approach.)

- Another advantage of this technique is that you get to spend some time with patients and their families while you perform the local anesthetic injection and the wide awake procedure. It provides a significant opportunity for patient education.

- Patients express greater overall satisfaction when you perform their procedure with the minimal pain method outlined in Chapter 5.

It may seem like a giant leap of faith to perform your cases with local anesthetic only. I have several suggestions for you if you are interested in using this technique.

DO SOME HOMEWORK

There are several excellent articles published describing the WALANT technique and medication dosages.[1-4] They are well worth your time to read, but their material is contained in greater detail in this book.

START SMALL

Don't schedule a Dupuytren's fasciectomy as your first WALANT case. I started with a small case: a trigger finger with sedation on standby and a tourniquet on the arm, but not inflated. Once you see that this works, you can progress to carpal tunnel releases and other procedures.

FOLLOW THE RULES

The published literature and this book describe the WALANT technique and local doses nicely: Do not try to innovate or create a new protocol in your early experience with the technique. When you use 1:100,000 epinephrine, the maximal vasoconstriction occurs approximately 26 minutes after an injection.[5] If you try to cut the waiting time short, you will be disappointed. That's why it is important to do the local injection in a preoperative holding area. Make certain you do the injection with the patient supine. This will help to minimize the vasovagal (fainting) events. Remember that the wound will not be completely dry. Although this will not be a significant problem, the wound will ooze somewhat initially.

DO A SITE VISIT

If you still have doubts about the benefits of WALANT, schedule a site visit with someone who is using the technique. I will admit that I was initially skeptical about this technique. However, once you see how the process works, including your increased efficiency and patient satisfaction, you won't go back to the old way of performing hand surgery.

WHY AND WHEN I USE THE WALANT TECHNIQUE

Günter Germann

I came from a classical background in hand surgery, with plexus blocks and general anesthesia with a bloodless tourniquet field. This and my work on cytokine release after tourniquet ischemia[1] made it almost irritating to see Dr. Lalonde first promoting the wide awake approach.[5]

- WALANT has now become an integral part of our hand surgical practice. A major advantage of the WALANT technique is that the patient can actively move his or her fingers so we are able to evaluate the functional result intraoperatively.

- Patient satisfaction is high, and results with flexor tendon repair and other operations can be better than with traditional techniques. (See Chapter 32, flexor tendon repair, Chapter 38, tenolysis, and Chapter 39, tendon transfer.)

- In the first cases, we did not wait long enough after injection of the local anesthetic. Patients had residual pain. Since we started waiting 30 minutes, we have not encountered this problem.

- Initially, we were not generous enough with the amount of local anesthetic. Changing that early in our practice eliminated patient discomfort.

- We feel that using a 27-gauge needle helps to decrease the pain of the injection.

- Today we use the WALANT approach whenever we think it is appropriate. Our experiences are promising, and the technique has stood the test of time.[6] However, we still have a number of patients who wish to have some sort of sedation so they will be "detached" from the surgical intervention. We provide that for those patients.

WALANT IS MY METHOD OF CHOICE FOR MUCH OF MY HAND SURGERY

Jason Wong

I was an early enthusiast of the WALANT technique because of my interest in improving outcomes in flexor tendon repair. I've subsequently applied the method to most hand procedures that I feel comfortable with and perform regularly.

- For flexor tendon surgery, this is the biggest positive change since the introduction of early true active motion. It is my method of choice.

- WALANT is not for the uninitiated, because it requires you to be comfortable performing hand surgery with a small amount of bleeding. You also have to be familiar with anatomic variations. Hence this technique is easier for experienced surgeons.

- I feel that the real merits lie in:
  - The ability to assess function on the table
  - Gaining access to operating rooms without the need for anesthesiology cover
  - The opportunity to communicate with and get to know your patients
  - Increased patient compliance; patients realize how much time and effort you have put into their surgery. They more readily keep their appointments and perform their subsequent hand therapy as instructed, as they have experienced it with you.
- I try to avoid WALANT procedures in:
  - Individuals who are very anxious and will undergo complex procedures
  - Patients having secondary or corrective surgery
  - Those with Raynaud's phenomenon, previous digital ischemia, or scleroderma
  - Very young children, except for straightforward amputation of accessory digits

ADDITIONAL CONSIDERATIONS

Donald H. Lalonde

The unlikely worst case scenario could be that you need to abandon WALANT because the patient is unable to tolerate it, or you run into unforeseen problems intraoperatively. That has never happened to me. However, if it did, I would simply cover the wound with a bandage or close the skin and finish the operation later or on another day with the patient under general anesthesia. This is not a terrible fallback position.

TRY THE TECHNIQUE FIRST WITH PATIENTS ASLEEP BUT WITHOUT A TOURNIQUET

As soon as possible after your anesthesiologist has the patient asleep or sedated, before you prepare and drape, inject the tumescent lidocaine and epinephrine solution as described in Chapter 4. After that injection, apply the safety net tourniquet that you will likely not inflate. By the time you scrub, prep, and drape the patient, the epinephrine will have had at least 5 to 10 minutes to work. The effect will not be as complete as if the epinephrine had 26 minutes to work, but you will still find the bleeding acceptable for good vision.

The wound will bleed a little when you cut the skin, but try to ignore this. Pull firmly on the Senn retractors and divide the transverse carpal ligament or A1 pulley. By the time you have done that, most of the bleeding will be drying up, and you will see that you have survived and managed quite well without a tourniquet. If you are able to wait 26 minutes before you make the first incision, you will have very little to cauterize at the end. I have not used cautery for trigger finger and carpal tunnel procedures in Saint John for 25 years.

WORKING WITH AN ANESTHESIOLOGIST

- If you are working with an anesthesiologist, ask him or her to use only propofol. Inject the lidocaine with epinephrine as soon as the propofol permits injection of pain-free local anesthetic. The anesthesiologist can stop all medication right after your injection and wake up the patient. This will give you the ability to perform intraoperative patient teaching (see Chapter 8) with a fully cooperative patient who can perform pain-free movement.

- Suggest that the anesthesia provider totally avoid opioids and amnestics to prevent nausea and allow the patient to remember your intraoperative advice.

- We try to avoid making an incision immediately after injection. We inject our patients in rooms outside the operating room, such as the postanesthesia care unit (recovery room). We do this so the wound site will bleed less when we make the first incision. It takes an average of 26 minutes for maximal vasoconstriction to peak after 1:100,000 epinephrine injection in humans.[5] Lidocaine also increases its numbing effect over that time.

- The numbness provided by lidocaine with epinephrine lasts an average of 5 hours in the hand[4] when we use median and ulnar nerve blocks as part of the tumescent local anesthesia. Numbness lasts an average of 10 hours as a digital block with epinephrine.[6] We inject one or two patients ahead of the one we are operating on so the lidocaine and epinephrine each have at least 26 minutes to take effect (see Chapter 14).

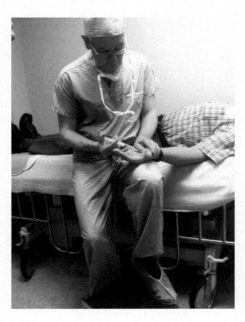

Injecting patients outside the main operating room in the patient holding area or in the recovery room on a stretcher helps to decrease the risk of the patient's fainting (see Chapter 6) and gives the lidocaine and epinephrine 26 minutes or more to work.

HEMOSTASIS

- We seldom use a cautery for WALANT surgery, but we have it available. At a concentration of 1:100,000, epinephrine produces very good hemostasis. Setting up a cautery with every case is a waste of time and money. If we encounter a larger vein, we clamp it with a hemostat and leave it to clot for a few minutes or tie it off.

- The higher the concentration of epinephrine, the better the hemostasis, and the longer the vasoconstriction will last.[7] However, 1:400,000 to 1:1,000,000[8] concentrations provide enough hemostasis that cautery is not required for most cases.

- Simply ignore the small amount of bleeding after the incisions and it will dry up. The time you will save by not having to cauterize bleeders after letting down a tourniquet will be worth it.

References

1. Lalonde DH, Wong A. Dosage of local anesthesia in wide awake hand surgery. J Hand Surg Am 38:2025, 2013.
2. Lalonde D, Martin A. Tumescent local anesthesia for hand surgery: improved results, cost effectiveness, and wide-awake patient satisfaction. Arch Plast Surg 41:312, 2014.
3. Lalonde D. Minimally invasive anesthesia in wide awake hand surgery. Hand Clin 30:1, 2014.
4. Chandran GJ, Chung B, Lalonde J, Lalonde DH. The hyperthermic effect of a distal volar forearm nerve block: a possible treatment of acute digital frostbite injuries? Plast Reconstr Surg 126:946, 2010.
5. McKee DE, Lalonde DH, Thoma A, Glennie DL, Hayward JE. Optimal time delay between epinephrine injection and incision to minimize bleeding. Plast Reconstr Surg 131:811, 2013.
6. Thomson CJ, Lalonde DH. Randomized double-blind comparison of duration of anesthesia among three commonly used agents in digital nerve block. Plast Reconstr Surg 118:429, 2006.
7. Fitzcharles-Bowe C, Denkler KA, Lalonde DH. Finger injection with high-dose (1:1000) epinephrine: does it cause finger necrosis and should it be treated? Hand (N Y) 2:5, 2007.
8. Prasetyono TO, Biben JA. One-per-mil tumescent technique for upper extremity surgeries: broadening the indication. J Hand Surg Am 39:3, 2014.

CHAPTER 14
SCHEDULING FIFTEEN OR MORE HAND SURGERY CASES PER DAY

Donald H. Lalonde

HOW TO BOOK A DAY OF FIFTEEN OR MORE ELECTIVE CASES

With good planning and coordination with staff, it is possible to schedule 15 or more elective cases per day that one surgeon, one nurse, and one receptionist can accomplish in the office or hospital minor procedure room in the clinic.

- For the first three cases, schedule simple procedures: carpal tunnel or trigger finger repairs. Ask the patients to come at 7:45 AM, 7:50 AM, and 7:55 AM.

- Schedule longer cases and trauma cases with less predictable lengths later in the day in the event that those procedures run overtime.

- Inject the first three patients with local anesthetic.

- Inject patients while they are lying down on a stretcher. They are less likely to faint (vasovagal reaction) if they are lying down.

- As soon as patients feel well after the injection, they can be asked to sit in a chair to liberate the stretcher so you can inject another patient. Two stretchers and an operating table to inject patients are ideal in the event you encounter a patient who faints and needs to remain lying down for a while. However, if necessary, one stretcher and one operating table will suffice for local anesthetic injections.

- After you inject the first three patients, complete their paperwork.

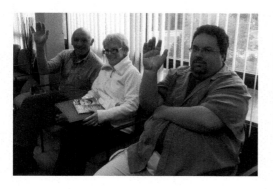

After we inject patients while they are lying down on a stretcher in the office, they sit up and wait at least 30 minutes for the lidocaine and epinephrine to work optimally. The setup is the same in the ambulatory clinic in the hospital. The patients with their hand up have had their injection.

- While you inject the first three patients and do their paperwork, the nurse sets up the first patient on the operating table and opens the tray of surgical instruments.

- We perform most clinic and office surgeries safely with field sterility, which greatly increases efficiency (see Chapter 10).

- After you finish the first operation, inject the fourth patient and do paperwork while the nurse sets up the tray for the second case and brings the second patient into the minor procedure room.

- The nurse can put on a pair of gloves and perform retraction if needed during part of the surgery. The rest of the time, the nurse circulates. You get your own instruments off the tray.

- Always try to inject one or two patients ahead of the one you are operating on so the lidocaine and epinephrine have at least 30 minutes to work optimally. It takes an average of 26 minutes for maximal vasoconstriction to peak after 1:100,000 epinephrine injection in humans.[1]

- Do not inject the patient and make an incision immediately after. The site will bleed less if you organize your time as described to allow an adequate interval for the epinephrine to work. The lidocaine component also increases its effect over 30 minutes and lasts over 4 hours in the hand when you block the median nerve as part of tumescent local anesthesia[2] (Chapter 18). Numbness in the finger lasts 10 hours when you inject lidocaine with epinephrine.[3] (See Chapter 1, Atlas, for specifics on injection placement, timing, and duration.)

- You can conduct most of your communication with the patient while you inject the local anesthetic and as you operate (see Chapter 8).

- If you are working with medical students or residents, first teach them how to give local anesthetic injections in a minimally painful fashion (have them read Chapter 5 and look at the videos first), and have the patients score their injection technique. When they amaze patients with minimal pain injections, the patients will be much more comfortable about allowing them to participate in the surgery under your direction.

- Clip 14-1 demonstrates that three carpal tunnel procedures can be performed per hour at a relaxed pace by one surgeon and one nurse.

Clip 14-1 Three carpal tunnel procedures performed per hour.

INTEGRATING PATIENT CONSULTATIONS FROM THE EMERGENCY DEPARTMENT AND TRAUMA SURGERY IN A HOSPITAL CLINIC

- We schedule our emergency department consultations to come to the hand surgery clinic in the hospital at 8 AM Mondays and Fridays, where we triage them and operate on those who need surgery (see hospital setup clips in Chapter 16).

- When we see a list of patients who arrive from the emergency department for consultation, we do not know which ones will need surgery. When we evaluate a patient who needs surgery, we go ahead and inject that patient at the end of the consultation. If necessary, he or she can wait for 1 or 2 hours after we inject the local anesthetic, and it will not wear off. After we finish our nonsurgical consultations, we perform surgeries on those patients who need it.

- If we know ahead of time that there are trauma patients requiring surgery who are coming to our clinic, we schedule them to come an hour before the end of the clinic consultation patients. This allows the surgical patients an hour in which the local anesthetic can take effect before we perform their surgery. In the meantime, we can finish seeing our clinic consultation patients.

References

1. McKee DE, Lalonde DH, Thoma A, Glennie DL, Hayward JE. Optimal time delay between epinephrine injection and incision to minimize bleeding. Plast Reconstr Surg 131:811, 2013.
2. Chandran GJ, Chung B, Lalonde J, Lalonde DH. The hyperthermic effect of a distal volar forearm nerve block: a possible treatment of acute digital frostbite injuries? Plast Reconstr Surg 126:946, 2010.
3. Thomson CJ, Lalonde DH. Randomized double-blind comparison of duration of anesthesia among three commonly used agents in digital nerve block. Plast Reconstr Surg 118:429, 2006.

CHAPTER 15
INTEGRATING HAND THERAPISTS INTO WALANT

Susan Kean, Amanda Higgins, Donald H. Lalonde

INCORPORATING HAND THERAPISTS INTO YOUR HAND SURGERY CLINIC

If you do not presently have hand therapists seeing patients with you full time in your hand surgery clinic, you should think about making that happen for at least a few hours per week. There are many advantages to this[1]:

1. You can educate each other so you both enhance your skills.

2. Verbal communication between you and the hand therapists will produce better patient outcomes in complex problems such as flexor tendon repair and reconstruction.

3. The patient will see that you are a team and will want to become an active participant in your efforts to produce the optimal outcome.

4. The patient will see that you value the therapist's opinion and thus will be more likely to listen to the therapist and comply with instructions.

5. In some systems such as ours, therapists can take over patient care from the surgeon and complete the care for many hand problems. This frees up the surgeon's time, and the therapist can provide excellent ongoing one-on-one care.

6. If you begin performing WALANT hand surgery in your clinic, therapists can watch the surgery and assess the patients. In addition, therapists can educate the patient between the time of local anesthetic injection and surgery, as well as during the surgery itself. Clip 15-1 shows hand therapists engaging in preoperative therapy consultation between injection of local anesthetic and surgery for a flexor tendon repair in a 10-year-old girl.

Clip 15-1 Hand therapists in preoperative therapy consultation.

7. Therapists will waste a lot less time and avoid making judgment errors based on inadequate information because they could not communicate with the surgeon.

8. It will be easier for you to start doing early protected movement for finger fractures if the therapists see patients with you in the clinic (see Chapter 41).

HOW TO INTEGRATE HAND THERAPISTS INTO YOUR CLINICS AND WALANT PROCEDURES

- The surgeon must initiate the effort to integrate therapists into the clinic—because no one else will do it. You can begin by making appointments with the hospital and therapy administrators to get this process started.

- Arrange to talk to the key hospital administrators one at a time. Convince them that you need a hand therapist to come to your clinic for 1 hour once a week so you can see patients with complex hand conditions with him or her. You can schedule complex patients to arrive when the therapist is there so no time is wasted. We began this in our hospital 25 years ago. One hour became 2 hours; once a week became twice a week; one therapist became two therapists. We now have two or three therapists for 4 hours 3 days a week.

- We perform our WALANT hand minor trauma procedures in the clinic in one room while the therapists are working in another clinic room where they make orthoses (splints) and see patients (see Chapter 16 for a video of our clinic setup). These are primarily hand fractures and tendon and nerve lacerations. Major hand trauma is still handled in the main operating room.

- We ask the therapists to come into the clinic operating rooms to observe parts of procedures. They perform intraoperative patient assessment and education as required (see clips that follow) in between their splinting and consultation duties.

- Point out anatomic structures to the therapists, much as you would do with a medical student or resident. Demonstrate how reconstructed tendons and bones move or function during the surgery.

- Hand therapists will start to engage with the patient even before the surgery. Therapists can start patient education in the time after the local anesthetic injection while the surgeon is seeing other patients and waiting for the local anesthetic to take optimal effect. When they are familiar with your techniques, they can do a better job of educating your patients about what to expect after surgery. This will be even easier for them if they have seen you perform the surgery.

- Do not forget that the hand therapist is in the room! Talk with the therapist about what you are seeing or doing. This will help him or her to determine the best postoperative care.

ADVANTAGES FOR HAND THERAPISTS IN GENERAL

- They see live tissue and how it functions with active movement during surgery.

- They understand surgical technique because they have seen it first-hand, not just from hearing or reading about it.

- They can assess patient compliance and reliability before, during, and after the operation.

- There is real-time interaction between the surgeon and therapist, avoiding miscommunication about the outcome and treatment plan.

- This establishes the therapist in the "role of coach" to the patient.

ADVANTAGES FOR THE PATIENT

- An educated patient who has undergone wide awake hand surgery is aware of what happened during surgery and what he or she needs to do for a successful recovery.

- From the start, the patient becomes an active participant in the rehabilitation team with the surgeon and the therapist.

- The patient's intraoperative interaction places ownership for postoperative care squarely on his or her shoulders.

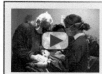

Clip 15-2 Patient watching structures being repaired.

ADVANTAGES FOR HAND THERAPY IN FLEXOR TENDON REPAIR

- See Chapter 32 for extensive discussions in both video and text on postoperative therapy of flexor tendon repair.

- In Clip 15-3 the surgeon and therapist teach the patient about the Saint John postoperative protocol during flexor tendon surgery.

- Therapists can see intraoperative full fist active flexion and extension testing of tendon integrity (no gapping) and glide-through pulleys at the time of surgery.

- The therapist can initiate communication regarding repair and the treatment protocol with the surgeon and patient before, during, and immediately after the surgery.

Clip 15-3 Intraoperatively the surgeon and therapist teach the patient about postoperative care.

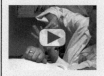

Clip 15-4 Therapist teaching a patient during flexor tendon repair surgery.

Clip 15-5 Allowing wrist extension and active flexion after flexor tendon repair.

- When therapists see full fist flexion and extension without gapping at surgery, they know that 3 days later the patient is unlikely to have gapping and rupture if he or she limits movement to half a fist. This helps therapists gain the increased confidence to move the repaired tendon early with true active movement for better results with less potential for rupture and tenolysis.[2] (See Chapter 32 for videos of up to half a fist of active movement.)

ADVANTAGES FOR HAND THERAPY IN EXTENSOR TENDON REPAIR

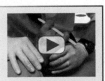

Clip 15-6 Relative motion extension splinting for extensor tendon repair.

- Seeing no gap at surgery with intraoperative testing of the repair with simulated relative motion extension splinting assures the surgeon and therapist that they can allow the patient an earlier return to work (as early as 3 to 5 days postoperatively) wearing a relative motion extension splint.[3]

- Watching the repaired hand move during surgery helps therapists decide whether they should incorporate the wrist component of relative motion extension splinting or not.[1]

- Therapists can see and assess the stress placed on the repair when they start early protected movement (see Chapters 35 and 36).

ADVANTAGES FOR HAND THERAPY IN FINGER FRACTURES

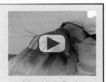

Clip 15-7 Early protected active motion after K-wired repair of finger fractures decided with the therapist during surgery.

- Therapists and surgeons are able to see how stable the reduced finger fractures are when they move after K-wire insertion at surgery. This increases confidence for both the surgeon and therapists to begin early protected active movement protocols after fixing finger fractures with K-wires[4] (Chapter 41).

- See Chapter 41 for extensive discussions in videos and text on early protected movement with hand therapy after K-wiring finger fractures. You can move fingers early, as you do with flexor tendon repairs.

- Watching active movement during surgery lets therapists and surgeons know whether K-wire placement interferes with joint motion.

- Seeing active movement during the surgery helps the surgeons and therapists decide what kind of splint to use to protect the fracture after surgery.

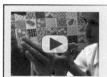

Clip 15-8 Therapist teaching early movement 3 days after K-wiring finger fractures.

References

1. Lalonde DH. How the wide awake approach is changing hand surgery and hand therapy: inaugural AAHS sponsored lecture at the ASHT meeting, San Diego, 2012. J Hand Therapy 26:175, 2013.
2. Higgins A, Lalonde DH, Bell M, McKee D, Lalonde JF. Avoiding flexor tendon repair rupture with intraoperative total active movement examination. Plast Reconstr Surg 126:941, 2010.
3. Merritt WH. Relative motion splint: active motion after extensor tendon injury and repair. J Hand Surg Am 39:1187, 2014.
4. Jones NF, Jupiter JB, Lalonde DH. Common fractures and dislocations of the hand. Plast Reconstr Surg 130:722e, 2012.
5. Burns MC, Derby B, Neumeister MW. Wyndell Merritt immediate controlled active motion (ICAM) protocol following extensor tendon repairs in zone IV-VII: review of literature, orthosis design, and case study-a multimedia article. Hand (N Y) 8:17, 2013.

CHAPTER 16

MINOR PROCEDURE ROOM SETUP

Donald H. Lalonde, Geoff Cook

With the advent of WALANT and field sterility, we perform most of our hand surgery in minor procedure rooms outside of the main operating room. In this chapter, we provide videos and descriptions of the minor procedure room setup in two hospitals and one surgeon's office where we perform these procedures in Saint John, New Brunswick, Canada.

PHYSICAL SPACE

A reception area with seating and a receptionist to manage this area is essential. After you inject patients with local anesthetic, most can go back to sit in the reception area to wait for their procedure with their families. This allows a half hour between injection of the local anesthetic and the onset of optimal numbing and epinephrine vasoconstriction.[1]

OUR FACILITIES IN SAINT JOHN, NEW BRUNSWICK, CANADA

We have performed wide awake hand surgery for more than 30 years in our facility with a relatively modest investment of money, space, equipment, and staffing for our accredited minor procedure rooms.

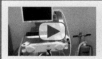

Clip 16-1 Clinic consultation and minor procedure room setup at the Saint John Regional Hospital.

Clip 16-2 Clinic consultation and minor procedure room setup at St. Joseph's Hospital.

Clip 16-3 Minor procedure accredited operating room at Dr. Lalonde's office.

MINOR PROCEDURE ROOMS

- Our office minor procedure room in Canada is accredited by the Canadian Association for Accreditation of Ambulatory Surgical Facilities (CAAASF), *http://caaasf.org,* for pure local anesthesia (no sedation).
- In the United States, as in Canada, you can have a minor procedure room in your office accredited for pure local anesthesia (no sedation)

by the American Association for Accreditation of Ambulatory Surgery Facilities (AAAASF), *http://www.aaaasf.org,* more easily and with much less cost than you would need for accreditation for performing procedures with sedation or general anesthesia.

- It is ideal to have two or more stretchers in addition to the procedure table on which to inject lying-down (supine) patients, but one is sufficient. We do injections with the patient lying down instead of sitting up to decrease the risk of fainting (see Chapter 6).

- In one of our hospitals, we have access to only one procedure room most of the time. In this situation, we inject patients on stretchers in other rooms down the hall. After we inject the local anesthetic, most patients can then sit with their relatives for 30 minutes or more before surgery while the local anesthetic achieves optimal numbing and vasoconstriction. If patients need to remain lying down because of fainting or other issues, we let them lie on their stretcher until we move them to the procedure room.

- All you really need in a procedure room is a stretcher that can be adjusted to the Trendelenburg position (head down, feet up), an arm board, and a good light (fixed or portable). All hospitals have these facilities.

- Cleaning staff wash the minor procedure room floors in the evening, but not between cases, unless there is an infection issue such as abscess drainage or a patient who has been identified as having a methicillin-resistant *Staphylococcus aureus* (MRSA) infection.

PERSONNEL

- In addition to the receptionist, only one nurse is required to help the surgeon for most simple cases such as carpal tunnels and trigger fingers.

- The nurse both circulates and assists. She puts on gloves only to hold retractors if and when necessary. The surgeon gets his own instruments off the tray. We get a second assistant for complex cases, such as fracture reduction.

- No recovery room or recovery personnel are required, since no sedation is given, which would require recovery. Patients just sit up and go home after the surgery.

EQUIPMENT

SURGICAL EQUIPMENT IN OUR MINOR PROCEDURE ROOM

- For minor hand surgery procedures such as carpal tunnel surgery, we use small drapes with a hole, or small sterile towels.

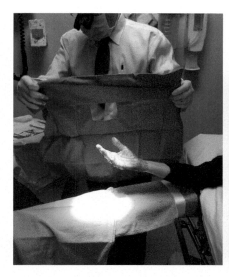
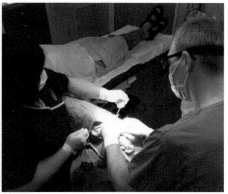

A typical Canadian minor procedure room setup with field sterility (see Chapter 10) for performing carpal tunnel surgery with one surgeon and one nurse assistant. The nurse puts on gloves only to hold retractors if and when necessary. The nurse both circulates and assists. The surgeon takes his own instruments off the tray. This is the way most Canadian carpal tunnel surgery is performed.[2]

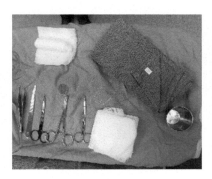

A basic instrument tray for carpal tunnel surgery includes scalpel handle, forceps, suture scissors, dissecting scissors, a needle holder, and a cup to hold the sterilizing liquid.

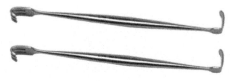

Two Senn retractors for carpal tunnel procedures. We open the Senn retractors separately.

- We use Desmarres (vein) retractors wrapped separately for trigger fingers and De Quervain surgery (see Chapter 21 for a photo of Desmarres retractors).

- Also wrapped separately, we keep periosteal elevators, skin hooks, hemostats, rongeurs, towel clips to reduce fractures, K-wires, curettes, and army-navy retractors for lacertus tunnel release.

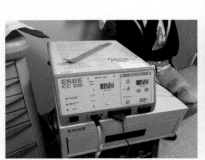
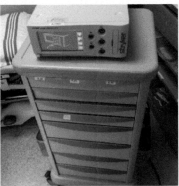

We have a cautery machine available in the minor procedure room but seldom use it. We also have an electric K-wire driver.

A low-radiation C-arm (such as the Hologic Fluoroscan InSight-FD Mini C-arm) is very valuable for diagnostic and therapeutic procedures. A radiation technologist is not required because of the low radiation produced by these types of devices.[3]

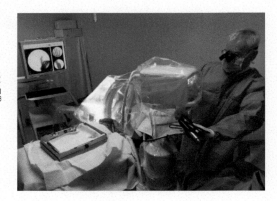

- We have sterile gowns and large drapes available when we choose to have augmented field sterility for cases such as open finger and hand fractures, and flexor tendon repairs. Sterile C-arm drapes are also available.

- We do have a tourniquet but seldom use it. We use a sterile ¼-inch Penrose drain for a tourniquet for some finger procedures such as nail bed work, schwannoma, or giant cell tumor excision.

- An ultrasound machine is also helpful for diagnostic and therapeutic purposes if possible. Sterile covers can be purchased for the ultrasound probe for intraoperative use.

HAND TRAUMA

- In many Canadian cities, most trauma surgery, such as K-wiring fractures and repairing lacerated tendons and nerves, happens in clinic minor procedure rooms. We operate at our convenience in daytime hours with field sterility (see Chapter 10).

- Our typical telephone discussion with the emergentologist is like this: "Thank you for your (Saturday night) call. I would be so grateful if you would kindly wash it out, close the skin, and we will be delighted to see the patient in the clinic Monday/Friday morning."

- It is ideal to have a clinic adjacent to the minor procedure room where we see most patients referred from the emergency department. Our emergentologists refer most of them to the hand surgery clinics 4 mornings a week. There we triage them into those who need surgery and those who do not. Patients requiring surgery can have it done right there in the minor procedure rooms the morning we see them.

OTHER FACILITIES NEAR THE MINOR PROCEDURE ROOMS

- It is ideal to have the hand therapists working in a room nearby (see Clip 16-1) so we can invite them into our minor procedure rooms to witness tendon and fracture surgery, educate patients during the surgery, and fabricate splints before or after the surgery (see Chapter 15).

PROCEDURES NOT PERFORMED IN MINOR PROCEDURE ROOMS

- For some procedures, we prefer doing WALANT in a formal operating room environment for full sterility or vital sign monitoring of the patient.

- Full sterility is more desirable when inserting foreign bodies such as plates or joint implants. We also use main OR full sterility for long procedures in relatively avascular areas, such as thumb basal joint arthroplasty, extensive tendon transfers, or secondary tendon reconstruction.

- If a patient has cardiac issues and monitoring is desirable, we use monitors for WALANT patients in the main operating room. We can also decrease the concentration of epinephrine to 1:400,000. It washes out faster and bleeds a little more but still provides excellent visualization.

References

1. McKee DE, Lalonde DH, Thoma A, Glennie DL, Hayward JE. Optimal time delay between epinephrine injection and incision to minimize bleeding. Plast Reconstr Surg 131:811, 2013.
2. Leblanc MR, Lalonde J, Lalonde DH. A detailed cost and efficiency analysis of performing carpal tunnel surgery in the main operating room versus the ambulatory setting in Canada. Hand (N Y) 2:173, 2007.
3. Thomson CJ, Lalonde DH. Measurement of radiation exposure over a one-year period from Fluoroscan mini C-arm imaging unit. Plast Reconstr Surg 119:1147, 2007.

Part III

SPECIFIC DETAILS OF HOW TO PERFORM
WIDE AWAKE HAND SURGERY FOR
COMMON OPERATIONS

CHAPTER 17
FINGER AND RAY AMPUTATION

Donald H. Lalonde

ADVANTAGES OF WALANT VERSUS SEDATION AND TOURNIQUET FOR FINGER AND RAY AMPUTATION

Losing a finger is a major event in a patient's life. You get a precious 1-hour opportunity during the surgery to educate the patient on what to expect for recovery and future hand function. This can go a long way toward helping the patient to adapt to the physical changes in the hand.

- The patient gets to see what you remove. For example, you can open up a destroyed finger after removing it and offer to show the damaged parts to the patient. If he or she wants to see it, we have found that the individual may better understand and accept why an attempt to salvage the finger never was going to work. This can help in the "grieving" process for the amputated part.

- Patients get to see that all of the remaining parts of their hand have a full range of active movement after the amputation, at the end of the operation. After patients recover from the pain and stiffness of surgery, they realize that with therapy they can regain full movement in the remaining fingers.

- All of the general advantages of wide awake hand surgery listed in Chapter 2 apply to both the surgeon and the patient.

WHERE TO INJECT THE LOCAL ANESTHETIC FOR FINGER AMPUTATION

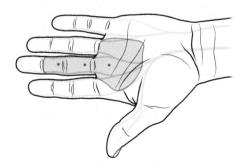

Palmar injections: Inject 10 ml of 1% lidocaine with 1:100,000 epinephrine (buffered with 1 ml of 8.4% sodium bicarbonate) in the most proximal palmer red injection point. Place the most proximal dorsal injection next, then inject 2 ml in the middle of each of the palmar proximal and middle phalanges in the subcutaneous fat. Performing the proximal dorsal injection before the two distal palmar injections gives it time to be blocked.

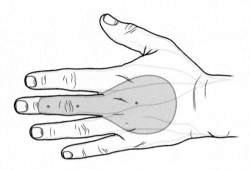

Dorsal injections: Inject 4 ml of 1% lidocaine with 1:100,000 epinephrine (buffered with 0.4 ml of 8.4% sodium bicarbonate) in the proximal red injection dot on the dorsal hand. Do the two palmar injections next, and then inject 2 ml in the middle of the dorsal proximal and middle phalanges in the subcutaneous fat.

- See Chapter 1, Atlas, for more illustrations of the anatomy of tumescent local anesthetic in the forearm, wrist, and hand.

MINIMALLY PAINFUL INJECTION OF LOCAL ANESTHETIC FOR FINGER AMPUTATION

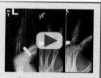

Clip 17-1 Local injection for proximal phalanx finger amputation.

- Inject just under the skin. There is no need to inject into the sheath; it would only add unnecessary pain. The local anesthetic will diffuse into the sheath.

- Inject the patient on a stretcher in a waiting area before he or she comes into the operating room a minimum of 30 minutes before surgery to allow the epinephrine to take optimal effect and to provide an adequately dry working field, as outlined in Chapters 4, 5, and 14.

- Inject the patient lying down to decrease the risk of fainting (see Chapter 6).

- To minimize the pain of injection, inject with a fine 27-gauge needle (not a 25-gauge) into the most proximal injection point (red dot).

- Ask the patient to look away. Press with a fingertip just proximal to the injection site before you put in the needle to add the sensory "noise" of pressure to decrease the pain.

- Insert the first needle perpendicularly into the subcutaneous fat. Stabilize the syringe with two hands to avoid pain from needle wobble until the skin needle site is numb. Inject the first visible 0.5 ml bleb and then pause. Wait 15 to 45 seconds until the patient tells you that all needle pain is gone. Inject the rest of the 10 ml slowly (over 3 minutes) without moving the needle.

- In this operation, inject the 10 ml in the most proximal part of the palm first, and then inject 4 ml in the most proximal part of the dorsal hand right after that. This will give at least a little time for the distal injection points to become numb before you inject them.

- The distal injections are for the epinephrine vasoconstriction effect; the skin is already numb from the proximal nerve blocks.

- There is no need to inject the palm if the finger amputation is at a more distal level than the proximal phalanx, as shown in Clip 17-2 of a finger amputation at the distal interphalangeal (DIP) joint.

- Clip 17-2 shows a SIMPLE block for a distal phalanx squamous cell cancer amputation of the distal phalanx of the long finger (see Chapters 1 and 5 for details of the SIMPLE block).

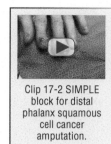

Clip 17-2 SIMPLE block for distal phalanx squamous cell cancer amputation.

WHERE TO INJECT THE LOCAL ANESTHETIC FOR RAY AMPUTATION

MINIMALLY PAINFUL INJECTION OF LOCAL ANESTHETIC FOR RAY AMPUTATION

- Inject 10 ml in the most proximal palmar red dot injection point in the subcutaneous fat and under the superficial palmar fascia without moving the needle. Then inject 10 ml in the most proximal red dorsal dot of in the subcutaneous fat over the dorsal proximal hand without moving the needle.

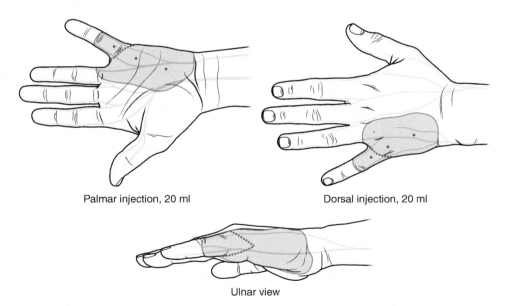

Palmar injection, 20 ml   Dorsal injection, 20 ml

Ulnar view

For ray amputation, inject 20 ml of 1% lidocaine with 1:100,000 (buffered with 10 ml lido/epi:1 ml of 8.4% sodium bicarbonate) epinephrine on each of the palmar and dorsal sides of the ray to be amputated, for a total of 40 ml.

- See Chapter 1, Atlas, for more illustrations of the anatomy of diffusion of tumescent local anesthetic in the forearm, wrist, and hand.

- If it is convenient, wait 15 to 30 minutes for the distal palmar and dorsal hand to get numb so the patient does not feel the distal injections.

- Then inject 8 ml in each of the palmar and dorsal central red dot injection points at the head of the metacarpal level in the subcutaneous fat between the digital nerves without moving the needle.

- Finally, inject 2 ml in the palmar and dorsal distal red dot injection points in the subcutaneous fat of the proximal phalanx.

- To decrease the pain of injections, use the other tips discussed in the finger amputation section above (also see Chapter 5).

TIPS AND TRICKS FOR PERFORMING FINGER AND RAY AMPUTATION WITH THE WIDE AWAKE APPROACH

- Wait 30 minutes after the last injection for the epinephrine to reach maximal vasoconstrictive effect, and then operate. Part of these 30 minutes can be spent bringing the patient into the operating room, prepping, draping, and other tasks.

- Warn the patient that he or she will hear sounds of bone and joint manipulation but will not feel pain. The patient may choose to listen to music on earphones.

- Get the patient to observe his or her hand going through a full range of active movement after you have cleansed the hand at the end of the operation. The patient will know that he or she can regain full movement again after the pain and stiffness of healing subside.

- Use the opportunity to educate the patient on postoperative care of the injured hand (see Chapter 8).

- Use the intraoperative opportunity while closing the skin to educate the patient on what to expect for recovery and future hand function. For example, you can discuss time out of work, phantom limb pain, etc. This can go a long way toward helping the patient adapt to his or her new hand.

CHAPTER 18
CARPAL TUNNEL DECOMPRESSION OF THE MEDIAN NERVE

Carolyn L. Kerrigan, Donald H. Lalonde, Shu Guo Xing, Jin Bo Tang

ADVANTAGES OF WALANT VERSUS SEDATION AND TOURNIQUET IN CARPAL TUNNEL DECOMPRESSION

- When you perform wide awake hand surgery, you do not have to deal with your patient's medical comorbidities, which would only be a problem if the patient has been sedated. It is safer for your patients to have no sedation. They just get up and go home after surgery, like when they have had a filling at the dentist.

- A major advantage of eliminating sedation for carpal tunnel surgery is that you do not need to perform the procedures in the main operating room. You can do all of your carpal tunnel surgeries in minor treatment rooms in the clinic outside the main operating room with evidence-based field sterility (see Chapter 10).

- You can easily perform 15 or more carpal tunnel releases in 1 day with only one nurse using field sterility in the office or clinic. You can also see consultation and recheck patients between operations (see Chapter 14).

- You avoid tourniquet let-down bleeding.

- You do not need to use a cautery, particularly if you inject the epinephrine 30 minutes before the first incision. We have not opened a cautery for over 25 years for carpal tunnel release. Hematoma has not been a problem, even in patients on anticoagulants.

- Your patient remains pain free with the median and ulnar nerve block for up to 5 hours using the technique described below.[1] Nausea and vomiting do not occur, because you have given the patient no perioperative narcotic agents.

- Although patients can "tolerate" 7 minutes of tourniquet control, they will not experience any tourniquet pain at all if you simply use epinephrine with the lidocaine. There is high-level published evidence that the tourniquet hurts twice as much as the injection of a local anesthetic in carpal tunnel surgery.[2,3] Patients appreciate the tourniquet-free experience.

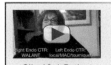

Clip 18-1 Patient impression of tourniquet with sedation versus WALANT for endoscopic carpal tunnel surgery.

- Dr. Kerrigan notes: "For years I used to do endoscopic carpal tunnel releases with a local anesthetic and with an upper arm tourniquet. I would often ask patients what bothered them the most, if anything, at the end of the procedure. The most common response I got was that the tourniquet was uncomfortable. Now (since I switched to the WALANT technique) when I ask the question, the most common response I get is, 'It really wasn't bad at all, not even as bad as going to the dentist.'"

- All of the general advantages listed in Chapter 2 apply to both the surgeon and the patient.

WHERE TO INJECT THE LOCAL ANESTHETIC FOR AN OPEN CARPAL TUNNEL RELEASE

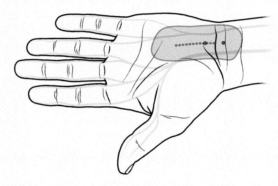

For carpal tunnel release, 20 ml of 1% lidocaine with 1:100,000 (buffered with 10 ml lido/epi:1 ml of 8.4% sodium bicarbonate) is injected.

- See Chapter 1, Atlas, for more illustrations of the anatomy of diffusion of tumescent local anesthetic in the forearm, wrist, and hand.

SPECIFICS OF MINIMALLY PAINFUL INJECTION OF LOCAL ANESTHETIC IN OPEN CARPAL TUNNEL RELEASE

Clip 18-2 A "hole-in-one" minimal pain local anesthetic injection for open carpal tunnel release.

- We inject the anesthetic solution a minimum of 30 minutes before surgery to allow the epinephrine to take optimal effect and provide an adequately dry working field.[4]

- We inject supine patients on stretchers in a waiting area to decrease the risk of their fainting (see Chapter 6).

- To minimize the pain of injection, use a fine 27-gauge needle (not a 25-gauge) into the most proximal red dot injection point.

- Ask the patient to look away. Press with a fingertip just proximal to the injection site before you put in the needle to add the sensory "noise" of touch and pressure to decrease the pain.

- Insert the first needle perpendicularly into the subcutaneous fat. Stabilize the syringe with two hands and have your thumb ready on the plunger to avoid the pain from needle wobble until the skin needle site is numb. Inject the first visible 0.5 ml bleb and then pause. Ask the patient to tell you when the needle pain is all gone. After he tells you the pain is gone, inject the rest of the first 10 ml slowly (over 2 minutes) without moving the needle.

- Ask the patient to tell you if he or she feels further episodes of pain during the injection so you can score your injection technique, as outlined in Chapter 5. If the patient feels pain twice, you score an eagle, three times a birdie, four times a bogie, and so on. It takes 5 minutes to perform the injection for a carpal tunnel release and consistently get a hole-in-one, where the patient feels only the stick of the first 27-gauge needle in the injection process.[5-7]

- Inject 10 ml of buffered 1% lidocaine with 1:100,000 epinephrine just ulnar to the palmaris longus at the proximal injection point, as shown in the figure on p. 130. This should be near the median nerve, but *never in the nerve.* Do not elicit paresthesias (electric shock feeling).

- The first 2 ml is injected just subcutaneous in the fat. Notice the location of small subcutaneous veins and avoid them.

- Advance slowly and more deeply to get under superficial fascia of the forearm to inject the remaining 8 ml for the median nerve block. This will also numb the ulnar nerve. If you are not under the forearm fascia, you may not block the nerve.

- After the initial 10 ml, come back to the subcutaneous plane with the needle tip and slowly infiltrate 10 ml from proximal to distal in an antegrade direction down the palm between the skin and the superficial palmar fascia. Blow the local anesthetic slowly ahead of the needle so there is always at least 1 cm of visible or palpable local anesthetic ahead of the sharp needle tip that the patient would feel if you advanced it into "live" nerves. Follow the rule of "Blow slow before you go." (See Chapter 5 for further tips on how to inject local anesthetic with minimal pain.)

- When reinserting the needle, do so into skin that is within 1 cm of clearly vasoconstricted white skin that has functioning lidocaine and epinephrine so the needle reinsertion is pain free.

- To avoid all pain in suturing the wound, be sure to have visible or palpable local anesthetic at least 1 cm on either side and 1 cm past the distal end of the palmar incision.

- You can also inject with a blunt-tipped cannula to increase the speed of painless injection compared with sharp needle tip injection (Clip 18-3 shows this blunt-tipped cannula injection for carpal tunnel surgery; also see Chapter 5). The blunt needle tip can push quickly with no pain past "live" unanesthetized nerves by gliding in the fat. Sharp

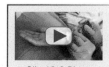

Clip 18-3 Blunt-tipped cannula injection of local anesthetic for carpal tunnel surgery.

needle tips will pierce nerves and cause pain if the local anesthetic is not bathing the nerve well ahead of the needle tip and if the operator is not moving slowly enough to let the local anesthetic work before the needle tip reaches the nerves. For this operation, insert a 37 mm long 27-gauge cannula into a needle hole created in numbed skin with a 25-gauge needle.

- Previous publications have documented the use of 10 ml for the median/ulnar nerve block and then another 10 ml in the palm.[6-8] Some surgeons think that 10 ml is an unnecessarily large volume for the median nerve block. Dalhousie New Brunswick medical students have recently performed a level I evidence study in which volunteers had bilateral median nerve blocks with 5 ml on one side and 10 ml on the other side. There were clearly more median nerve block failures in the 5 ml group than the 10 ml group (to be published).

- In some patients, the forearm fascia acts as a barrier to local anesthesia diffusion. If you only inject subcutaneously in the wrist, and do not have the needle under the forearm fascia, you may not get a median nerve block as the local may not penetrate the forearm fascia.

- Some people only inject under the skin with no intention of getting a median nerve block, and routinely successfully do carpal tunnel surgery under local this way. This works well. However, a possible disadvantage of this approach is that patients sometimes feel "electric jolts" when the live nerve is stimulated during the surgery.

- When you perform wide awake carpal and cubital (see Chapter 19) or lacertus tunnel (see Chapter 20) releases at the same time, simply decrease the concentration of the local anesthetic to 0.5% lidocaine with 1:200,000 epinephrine. For a cubital tunnel release, inject 60 ml at the elbow, as described in Chapter 19, and 20 ml in the hand for the carpal tunnel. For a lacertus tunnel release, inject 30 ml over the median nerve at the elbow, as described in Chapter 20, and 20 ml in the carpal tunnel.

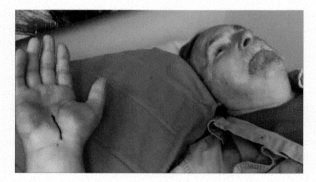

A comfortable position for the patient when performing an injection for a carpal tunnel release with local anesthetic is with the hand beside the patient's head on the pillow (elbow flexed).

WHERE TO INJECT THE LOCAL ANESTHETIC FOR AN ENDOSCOPIC CARPAL TUNNEL RELEASE

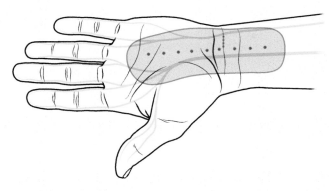

For an endoscopic carpal tunnel release procedure, 20 ml of 1% lidocaine with 1:100,000 epineph-rine (buffered with 10 ml lido/epi:1 ml of 8.4% sodium bicarbonate) is injected.

- See Chapter 1, Atlas, for more illustrations of the anatomy of diffusion of tumescent local anesthetic in the forearm, wrist, and hand.

SPECIFICS OF MINIMALLY PAINFUL INJECTION OF LOCAL ANESTHETIC IN ENDOSCOPIC CARPAL TUNNEL RELEASE

Carolyn L. Kerrigan

- After injecting a skin wheal, inject a further 2 to 3 ml of the local anesthetic solution under the forearm fascia 5 to 6 cm proximal to the wrist crease to block the median nerve.

- Inject 7 to 8 ml subcutaneously at three or four points from this first proximal forearm point to the wrist crease. The three or four forearm injection points will be 1 to 1.5 cm apart. Always reinsert the needle in a place where there is clearly visible tumescent local anesthetic underneath the skin, and where it has had time to work. In this way, the patient will only feel the single first stick of a 27-gauge needle for pain throughout the whole injection and operation.

- Staying subcutaneous (instead of subfascial) for the final forearm 7 to 8 ml of solution prevents flooding the endoscopic field with too much water which could impede visibility.

- The final 10 ml is injected subcutaneously in the palm from the wrist crease to the distal end of the transverse carpal ligament.

- The injection takes longer than the procedure, but the patients are amazed at how little pain they feel when it is performed this way.

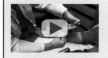

Clip 18-4 Injecting local anesthetic for endoscopic carpal tunnel release.

TIPS AND TRICKS FOR PERFORMING OPEN CARPAL TUNNEL PROCEDURES WITH THE WIDE AWAKE APPROACH

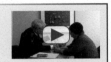

Clip 18-5 Patient consultation for carpal tunnel surgery.

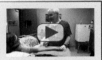

Clip 18-6 Advising the patient after injection of local anesthetic for carpal tunnel release.

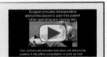

Clip 18-7 Intraoperative advice to the patient during carpal tunnel surgery.

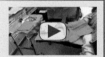

Clip 18-8 Field sterility setup for open carpal tunnel release.

- Managing patient expectations of WALANT carpal tunnel surgery begins with a calm, matter-of-fact approach about WALANT during the consultation.

- You can educate the patient during the local anesthetic injection (5 minutes) and during the surgery. This gives you 10 to 15 minutes of patient education time, which will decrease your complication rate and decrease the time you have to spend educating the patient in the office (see Chapter 8).

- For another video and additional discussion about giving intraoperative advice during carpal tunnel surgery, see Chapter 8.

- Inject two to four patients with local anesthetic outside the operating room before operating on the first one. This will give at least half an hour for the local anesthetic to work on these waiting patients, both for lidocaine numbing and for epinephrine vasoconstriction. It takes 26 minutes to achieve peak vasoconstriction in humans after 1:100,000 epinephrine injection (level I evidence).[4]

- After you inject the first patient, he or she will usually feel well enough to go sit in the waiting area with their injected arm raised until their surgery. You can then inject the second patient, then the third one. Then you can perform the surgery on the first one. While the nurse turns over the room after the first procedure, you can inject the fourth patient.

- In Canada, most carpal tunnel procedures are performed with field sterility in the manner shown in Clip 18-8. The cost is much less, and the patient convenience and satisfaction are much higher with field sterility outside the main operating room than with full sterility in the main operating room (see Chapter 10).

- Field sterility permits one hand surgeon and one nurse to perform 15 or more carpal tunnel procedures per day at a very leisurely pace (see Chapter 14).

- Get your assistant to pull very firmly on the Senn retractors to decrease the little bleeding that sometimes occurs, especially if the patient is hypertensive or receiving anticoagulants.

- *Never cut or suture where the skin is not white.* If there are no epinephrine molecules there causing vasoconstriction, there will likely not be any lidocaine molecules there either.

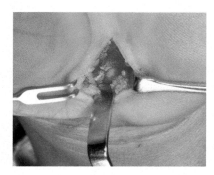

With WALANT, visibility is good with little bleeding, even with a 2 to 3 cm incision (Shu Guo Xing and Jin Bo Tang).

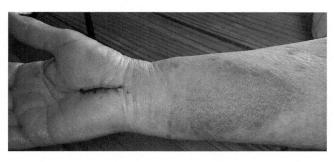

Early bruising with 10 ml of local anesthetic injected in the wrist can appear red and may make patients think they have an infection. This was not an infection but a bruise seen the day after surgery.

- Clip 18-9 shows carpal tunnel surgery, which includes prepping, draping, the operation, intraoperative advice, and a bandage for the open approach.

- Offer patients a guided tour of their carpal tunnel surgery. Many will accept and be delighted that they were given the opportunity to experience seeing the inside of their hand.

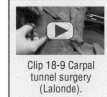

Clip 18-9 Carpal tunnel surgery (Lalonde).

IF YOU ARE WORKING WITH AN ANESTHESIOLOGIST

- Ask him or her to use only propofol. Inject the lidocaine with epinephrine as soon as the propofol permits pain-free injection of local anesthetic. The anesthesiologist can then wake the patient right away while you are scrubbing, prepping, and draping so you can get the benefit of intraoperative patient teaching (see Chapter 8). This will give the epinephrine a little time to become more effective. Suggest that the anesthesia provider avoid administering opiates and amnestics to prevent nausea and permit the patient to remember your intraoperative advice.

TIPS AND TRICKS FOR PERFORMING ENDOSCOPIC CARPAL TUNNEL SURGERY WITH THE WIDE AWAKE APPROACH

Carolyn L. Kerrigan

Clip 18-10
Endoscopic carpal
tunnel surgery.

I have been performing endoscopic carpal tunnel releases since 1991. Before I discontinued the use of a tourniquet, my conversion rate to an open procedure was 1 of 80 consecutive cases. I have done just over 80 WALANT cases, with a higher conversion rate during my learning curve. I have had eight conversions, mostly because of a lack of complete division of the distal margin of the transverse carpal ligament on palpation of the canal after I withdrew the scope. When I reintroduce the scope in this setting, the bleeding makes it difficult to see safely, and I have had to convert to an open approach. Most recently, I have made extra efforts to fully divide the most distal edge of the ligament and thus avoided the need for reintroduction of the scope after palpation with a dilator. The conversion approach has not required a full open exposure but rather a short counterincision in the palm, much like what one would make for a two-portal approach.

- Waiting at least 20 minutes on a timer is important, because this will result in a more profound anesthesia for the patient and visible blanching of the surgical site. The latter is important to minimize bleeding or oozing at the surgical site and into the endoscopic field.

- The greatest bleeding problems come from the incision site if you cut a superficial vein, which can then ooze into the wound and even into the scope device when you introduce it. Being cautious to avoid those superficial bleeders is extremely helpful to obviate that problem. The transverse carpal ligament itself is very avascular, and there will not be many problems with bleeding from the ligament itself.

References

1. Chandran GJ, Chung B, Lalonde J, Lalonde DH. The hyperthermic effect of a distal volar forearm nerve block: a possible treatment of acute digital frostbite injuries? Plast Reconstr Surg 126:946, 2010.
2. Braithwaite BD, Robinson GJ, Burge PD. Haemostasis during carpal tunnel release under local anaesthesia: a controlled comparison of a tourniquet and adrenaline infiltration. J Hand Surg Br 18:184, 1993.
3. Ralte P, Selvan D, Morapudi S, Kumar G, Waseem M. Haemostasis in open carpal tunnel release: tourniquet vs local anaesthetic and adrenaline. Open Orthop J 4:234, 2010.
4. McKee DE, Lalonde DH, Thoma A, Glennie DL, Hayward JE. Optimal time delay between epinephrine injection and incision to minimize bleeding. Plast Reconstr Surg 131:811, 2013.
5. Lalonde DH, Wong A. Local anesthetics: what's new in minimal pain injection and best evidence in pain control? Plast Reconstr Surg 134(4 Suppl 2):40S, 2014.
6. Lalonde DH. "Hole-in-one" local anesthesia for wide awake carpal tunnel surgery. Plast Reconstr Surg 126:1642, 2010.
7. Farhangkhoee H, Lalonde J, Lalonde DH. Teaching medical students and residents how to inject local anesthesia almost painlessly. Can J Plast Surg 20:169, 2012.
8. Lalonde DH, Wong A. Dosage of local anesthesia in wide awake hand surgery. J Hand Surg Am 38:2025, 2013.

CHAPTER 19

CUBITAL TUNNEL DECOMPRESSION OF THE ULNAR NERVE

Donald H. Lalonde, Alistair Phillips

ADVANTAGES OF WALANT VERSUS SEDATION AND TOURNIQUET IN CUBITAL TUNNEL DECOMPRESSION SURGERY

- Positioning patients with their elbow above their head is much easier for your access as the surgeon. The anesthesiologist and his or her equipment will not be occupying your valuable surgical access space.

- There is no tourniquet, so you have much easier access to the proximal incision.

- Patients can position themselves comfortably so the elbow and the shoulder are not sore during the surgery. They do not wake up from general anesthesia with shoulder pain that we caused by putting their shoulder in a position it does not like.

- You can see whether the ulnar nerve subluxates with active movement by watching patients actively flex and extend the elbow through a full range of motion before you close the skin. If the nerve subluxates, you can transpose it if required.

- You can perform cubital tunnel decompression with field sterility or augmented field sterility (see Chapter 10).

- All of the general advantages listed in Chapter 2 apply to both the surgeon and the patient.

Clip 19-1 Checking for ulnar nerve subluxation with active movement during surgery.

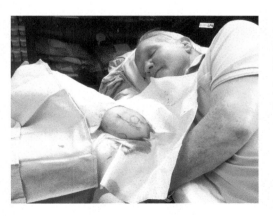

This patient with a stiff elbow and a sore shoulder has been placed in a comfortable position for a cubital tunnel release. We negotiated different positions until he found this one worked best to accommodate his stiff elbow and sore shoulder from old injuries.

WHERE TO INJECT THE LOCAL ANESTHETIC FOR CUBITAL TUNNEL DECOMPRESSION

Inject 60 ml of 0.5% lidocaine with 1:200,000 epinephrine buffered with 3 ml of 8.4% sodium bicarbonate for a ratio of 10 ml lido/epi:1 ml of 8.4% sodium bicarbonate.

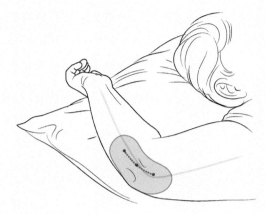

- See Chapter 1, Atlas, for more illustrations of the anatomy of diffusion of tumescent local anesthetic in the forearm, wrist, and hand.

SPECIFICS OF MINIMALLY PAINFUL INJECTION OF LOCAL ANESTHETIC FOR CUBITAL TUNNEL DECOMPRESSION

Clip 19-2 How to inject local anesthetic for cubital tunnel release at the elbow.

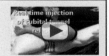

Clip 19-3 Real-time injection of local anesthetic for cubital tunnel release.

- Inject 20 ml subcutaneously in the most proximal part of the incision, followed by 20 ml in the middle of the incision, and then 20 ml at the end of the incision.

- Inject the anesthetic solution a minimum of 30 minutes before surgery to allow the epinephrine to take optimal effect and provide an adequately dry working field.

- We inject supine patients on stretchers in a waiting area to decrease the risk of their fainting (see Chapter 6).

- To minimize pain of injection, start with a fine 27-gauge needle (not a 25-gauge) into the most proximal injection point (red dot).

- Ask the patient to look away. Press with a fingertip just proximal to the injection site before you put in the needle to add the sensory "noise" of touch pressure to decrease the pain.

- Mix 30 ml of 1% lidocaine with 3 ml of 8.4% bicarbonate into a 50 ml bag of saline solution that contains only 30 ml. (You remove 20 ml from the 50 ml bag before adding the lidocaine.) This gives you 63 ml of 0.5% lidocaine with 1:200,000 epinephrine buffered 10:1 with 8.4% sodium bicarbonate.

- Insert the first needle perpendicularly into the subcutaneous fat. Stabilize the syringe with two hands to avoid causing pain from needle wobble until the skin needle site is numb. Inject the first visible 0.5 ml bleb and then pause. Wait 15 to 45 seconds until the patient tells you that all needle pain is gone. Inject the rest of the first 10 ml slowly (over 2 minutes) without moving the needle.

- Inject 20 ml at the proximal injection point of the incision, 20 ml at the middle injection point, and 20 ml at the distal injection point. Always reinsert injection needles into an area with 1 cm of blanched skin around it to ensure that needle reinsertion does not hurt.

- Inject just under the skin. There is no need to inject into the cubital tunnel; it would only add unnecessary pain. The local anesthetic will diffuse into the tunnel.

- If you want to perform endoscopic cubital tunnel decompression that goes farther distally in the forearm, you can inject another 20 ml or more distally in the forearm so that you have at least 2 cm of palpable or visible local anesthetic beyond your area of dissection.

- For those who prefer anterior transposition, the soft tissue in the new nerve path will need to be more extensively flooded with another 20 ml of local anesthetic. The image on p. 138 shows local anesthetic injection for simple cubital tunnel release.

- We have not worked out the technique for submuscular transposition at this time, since we do not do that operation. You would likely need to inject beneath the deep forearm fascia to accomplish that operation as a wide awake procedure.

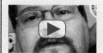

Clip 19-4 Injecting for both cubital tunnel and carpal tunnel release in the same operation.

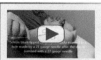

Clip 19-5 57 mm blunt-tipped 22-gauge cannula injection of local anesthetic for cubital tunnel release.

TIPS AND TRICKS FOR PERFORMING CUBITAL TUNNEL DECOMPRESSION WITH THE WIDE AWAKE APPROACH

- Many patients have a sore shoulder and wake up from general anesthesia with more shoulder pain after cubital tunnel release. When you perform an awake procedure, you can adjust their position for local anesthetic injection and surgery so you do not worsen their shoulder problem.

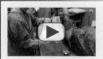

Clip 19-6 Prepping and draping for a WALANT cubital tunnel ulnar nerve release.

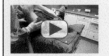

Clip 19-7 Cubital tunnel surgery with WALANT.

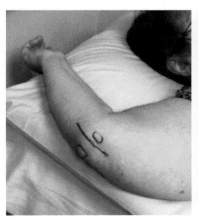
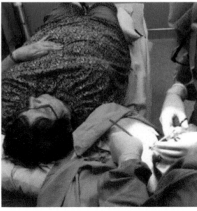

The elbow and shoulder are positioned at 90 degrees for injection of local anesthetic and surgery.

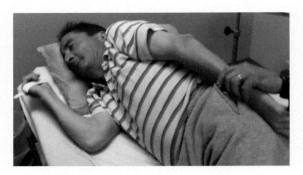

The surgery can be performed from behind with the patient on his side if he cannot abduct the shoulder.

- When the elbow is flexed, the nerve is tight in the canal, and there is less space to get your scissors in to open the roof of the canal. Ask the patient to extend the elbow until that maneuver is easy, then return the arm to elbow flexion. The awake cooperative patient makes this easy.

- Whether you use four towels with field sterility or half sheets for enhanced field sterility or full sterility, apply the drapes loosely enough to allow active full elbow flexion and extension.

- If we perform carpal tunnel release and cubital tunnel release at the same time, we inject the cubital tunnel with local anesthetic first and operate on it after the carpal tunnel release. This gives the epinephrine longer to work at the cubital tunnel, where hemostasis is more important.

- We do not routinely need cautery for cubital tunnel release, because we wait at least half an hour for the epinephrine to work. An hour is even better.

- After cubital tunnel release, get the patient to actively flex and extend the elbow to see if the nerve is subluxating. If you feel that a subluxating nerve will be a problem for the patient, you can tack it anteriorly on the forearm fascia as in anterior transposition.

CHAPTER 20

LACERTUS SYNDROME: MEDIAN NERVE RELEASE AT THE ELBOW

Elisabet Hagert, Donald H. Lalonde

Lacertus syndrome is characterized by compression of the median nerve under the lacertus fibrosus (bicipital aponeurosis) at the elbow. You can easily release this with good results in the right patients, as described in Clip 20-1. It is a simple procedure, similar to carpal tunnel release with WALANT.

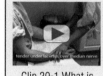

Clip 20-1 What is lacertus syndrome?

You make the diagnosis of lacertus syndrome on a clinical examination triad consisting of:

1. Weakness in the flexor carpi radialis (FCR), flexor pollicis longus (FPL), and flexor digitorum profundus muscles of the index finger (FDP2)

2. Pain over the median nerve at the medial edge of the lacertus fibrosus[1]

3. A positive scratch collapse test over the median nerve at the elbow

Clip 20-2 demonstrates clinical examination of lacertus syndrome showing weakness of FCR, FDP2, FPL, tenderness under lacertus fibrosis, and positive scratch collapse test.

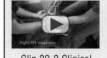

Clip 20-2 Clinical examination of lacertus syndrome.

- Although less prominent than motor signs, sensory symptoms in the median nerve distribution are present in some patients, especially in the palmar cutaneous branch distribution.

- Consider this diagnosis if patients complain of weakness or numbness in the palmar cutaneous distribution, or after failed carpal tunnel release.

- You will not make this diagnosis with nerve conduction studies. You make the diagnosis of lacertus syndrome through a history and a thorough physical motor examination.[2]

ADVANTAGES OF WALANT VERSUS SEDATION AND TOURNIQUET IN MEDIAN NERVE RELEASE AT THE ELBOW

- You can see that you have solved your patient's problem by watching him get the power back to his FPL, FDP2, and FCR on the operating table before you close the skin, as shown in four videos in this chapter.

- Your patient can see that you have solved his problem when he watches power return to his FPL, FDP2, and FCR on the operating table.

- Your fingertip can feel the superficialis sling actively flex over the median nerve inside the wound. You ask the patient to flex the long and ring fingers and feel the effect on the superficialis sling. You can choose to divide it if you feel it is a problem.

- All of the general advantages listed in Chapter 2 apply to both the surgeon and the patient.

WHERE TO INJECT THE LOCAL ANESTHETIC FOR LACERTUS TUNNEL RELEASE AT THE ELBOW

Inject at least 30 ml of 1% lidocaine with epinephrine 1:100,000 (available in North America) or 1:200,000 (available in Sweden) with 3 ml 8.4% sodium bicarbonate solution.

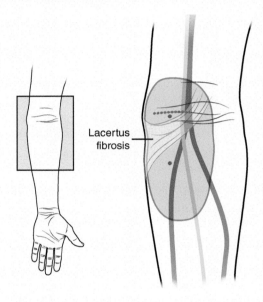

Lacertus fibrosis

- See Chapter 1, Atlas, for more illustrations of the anatomy of diffusion of tumescent local anesthetic in the forearm, wrist, and hand.

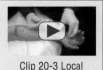

Clip 20-3 Local anesthetic injection for lacertus and carpal tunnel release.

SPECIFICS OF MINIMAL PAIN INJECTION OF LOCAL ANESTHETIC IN LACERTUS TUNNEL RELEASE AT THE ELBOW

- Inject in the fat just under the skin and superficial fascia from proximal to distal. There is no need to inject under the deep forearm muscle fascia. The goal is to leave the median nerve motor branches unanesthetized so you can test muscle power after you divide the lacertus.

- We inject the anesthetic solution a minimum of 30 minutes before surgery to allow the epinephrine to take optimal effect and provide an adequately dry working field,[3] as outlined in Chapter 4.

- We inject supine patients lying down on stretchers in a waiting area to decrease the risk of fainting (see Chapter 6).

- Since the skin on the volar aspect of the elbow is quite thin and elastic, pinch it lightly and insert the needle into the pinched and elevated skin to add the sensory "noise" of pressure to decrease the pain from the first needle insertion. You can also move the skin into the needle tip. Ask the patient to look away.

- Slowly inject to flood the incision area, and then advance obliquely to cover the course of the median nerve over a distance of at least 10 cm.

- To minimize pain of injection, start with a fine 27-gauge needle (not a 25-gauge) into the most proximal injection point (red dot).

- Inject the rest of the first 10 ml slowly (over 2 minutes) without moving the needle.

- Continue injecting from proximal to distal, blowing the local anesthetic slowly ahead of the needle. There should always be at least 1 cm of visible or palpable local anesthetic ahead of the sharp needle tip that would hurt the patient if you advanced it into "live" nerves. "Blow slow before you go." (See Chapter 5 for further tips on how to inject the local anesthetic with minimal pain.)

- Reinsert the needle farther distally into skin that is within 1 cm of clearly white and vasoconstricted tissue. If the epinephrine is working, so is the lidocaine. Needle reinsertion will not hurt.

- The more volume you inject, the greater the odds that no additional anesthetic will be required after you start to dissect. Try to avoid the need to "top-up" the anesthetic. The usual culprit is insufficient volume of tumescent local anesthetic.

- The anesthesia should cover the area between the medial epicondyle and biceps tendon, as well as distally past the lacertus fibrosus and the superficialis sling.

IF YOU ARE WORKING WITH AN ANESTHESIOLOGIST

- Ask him or her to use only propofol. Inject the lidocaine with epinephrine as soon as the propofol permits injection of pain-free local anesthetic. The anesthesiologist can then wake the patient right away while you are scrubbing, prepping, and draping. This will give you the benefit of intraoperative patient teaching (see Chapter 8) and fully cooperative pain-free movement. This will also allow a little time for the epinephrine to become more effective. Suggest that the anesthesia provider avoid administering opiates and amnestics to prevent nausea and permit the patient to remember your intraoperative advice.

TIPS AND TRICKS FOR PERFORMING LACERTUS TUNNEL RELEASE AT THE ELBOW WITH THE WIDE AWAKE APPROACH

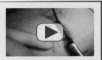

Clip 20-4 Surgical release of lacertus fibrosus by Dr. Elisabet Hagert.

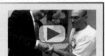

Clip 20-5 Lacertus and carpal tunnel injection and surgery by Dr. Don Lalonde.

- Resisted active elbow flexion during the surgery helps identify the biceps and lacertus fibrosus with your fingertip in the wound.

- In this condition, the brachial artery is frequently not palpable with a finger in the wound before you cut the thickened lacertus. After lacertus release, the brachial artery should be easily palpable from above the elbow to past the superficialis sling.

- When manipulating the lacertus, warn the patient that he or she may feel pressure.

- Be careful not to touch the median nerve, because the patient may feel unnecessary paresthesias. However, it may be helpful to warn the patient that he or she may feel a temporary pain akin to an "electrical current" out into the forearm and/or hand and that this is not dangerous. It just means that you are releasing the nerve.

- Once you have divided the lacertus fibrosus and released the median nerve, carefully let your finger slide distally and proximally over the nerve to rule out other compression points. If there is doubt as to possible entrapment of the median nerve at the superficialis sling, ask the patient to flex the ring and then the long fingers while you palpate at the level of the superficialis arcade. If you feel a constriction, consider releasing the superficialis arcade through a separate small transverse skin incision. You have already numbed this area.

- When you have adequately released the nerve, test the strength of the FPL and FDP2 to check for immediate improvement (see Clips 20-1 and 20-4). Ask patients to look at their hand as you test the strength, so they can see the action in the thumb and index finger. You can cover the wound with a towel if they do not want to see it. Patients will be pleased to see the power of their thumb and index finger return.

References

1. Hagert E. Clinical diagnosis and wide-awake surgical treatment of proximal median nerve entrapment at the elbow: a prospective study. Hand (N Y) 8:41, 2013.
2. Hagert CG, Hagert E. Manual muscle testing—a clinical examination technique for diagnosing focal neuropathies in the upper extremity. In Slutsky DJ, ed. Upper Extremity Nerve Repair: Tips and Techniques. A Master Skills Publication. Rosemont, IL: American Society for Surgery of the Hand, 2008.
3. McKee DE, Lalonde DH, Thoma A, Glennie DL, Hayward JE. Optimal time delay between epinephrine injection and incision to minimize bleeding. Plast Reconstr Surg 131:811, 2013.

CHAPTER 21

TRIGGER FINGER

Donald H. Lalonde

ADVANTAGES OF WALANT VERSUS SEDATION AND TOURNIQUET IN TRIGGER FINGER SURGERY

- Patients are able to see that the triggering action is gone as they watch themselves moving their fingers through a full range of motion before skin closure. They can see and anticipate that their hand will work well once they get past the postoperative discomfort and stiffness.

- You only need to divide the part of the pulley that is required to solve the problem as seen by active flexion, not the entire A1 pulley.

- After you release the pulley, you will occasionally see a band of fibrous tissue proximal to the pulley still causing triggering with active movement. You can release it and verify that you have solved the problem with full active flexion.

- A major advantage of eliminating sedation for trigger finger surgery is that you do not need to perform the procedure in the main operating room. We perform all trigger finger procedures in minor treatment rooms in the clinic outside the main operating room with field sterility (see Chapter 10).

- Many of these patients have diabetes, and because no sedation is given, you do not have to deal with their medical comorbidities, which are only a problem with sedation.

- You can easily perform 15 or more carpal tunnel releases mixed with trigger finger procedures in 1 day with only one nurse with field sterility in the office or clinic. You can also see consultation and recheck patients between operations (see Chapter 14).

- Although patients can "tolerate" 7 minutes of tourniquet use, they don't have to have any tourniquet pain at all if you simply use epinephrine with the lidocaine solution. There is ample high-level evidence that the tourniquet hurts twice as much as the local anesthetic injection in carpal tunnel surgery.[1,2] Patients appreciate the tourniquet-free experience.

- You avoid tourniquet let-down bleeding.

- You do not need cautery, particularly if you inject the lidocaine-epinephrine solution half an hour before you make an incision. We have not opened a cautery for 25 years for trigger fingers, and hematoma has not been a problem, even in patients receiving anticoagulants.

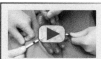

Clip 21-1 Trigger finger and thumb injection and surgery overview.

- Your patients remain pain free for at least 3 to 5 hours using the technique described below.
- There is no nausea and vomiting.
- All of the general advantages listed in Chapter 2 apply to both the surgeon and the patient.

WHERE TO INJECT THE LOCAL ANESTHETIC FOR TRIGGER FINGER AND TRIGGER THUMB

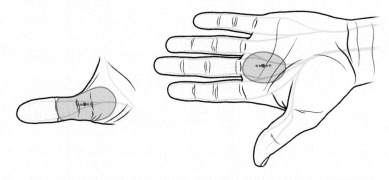

Inject 4 ml of 1% lidocaine with 1:100,000 epinephrine (buffered with 10 ml lido/epi:1 ml of 8.4% sodium bicarbonate) under the skin at the red injection dot site.

- See Chapter 1, Atlas, for more illustrations of the anatomy of diffusion of tumescent local anesthetic in the forearm, wrist, and hand.

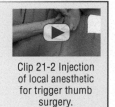

Clip 21-2 Injection of local anesthetic for trigger thumb surgery.

SPECIFICS OF MINIMALLY PAINFUL INJECTION OF LOCAL ANESTHETIC FOR TRIGGER FINGER SURGERY

- Inject just under the skin. There is no need to inject into the sheath; this would only add unnecessary pain. The local anesthetic will diffuse into the sheath.
- If you inject into the sheath, the local anesthetic will diffuse up the sheath into the whole finger or thumb. With enough pressure, the sheath will "explode" or burst. This will cause pain and send the epinephrine and lidocaine to the very end of the digit. This can cause a white fingertip. As with almost all white fingertips, it will eventually pink up. However, phentolamine can be injected to reverse the vasoconstriction (see Chapter 3).

- Inject the anesthetic solution a minimum of 30 minutes before surgery to allow the epinephrine to take optimal effect and provide an adequately dry working field, as outlined in Chapters 4 and 14.

- We inject supine patients lying down on stretchers to decrease the risk of their fainting (see Chapter 6).

- To minimize the pain of injection, start with a fine 27-gauge needle (not a 25-gauge).

- Ask the patient to look away. Press with a fingertip just proximal to the injection site before you put in the needle to add the sensory "noise" of pressure to decrease the pain.

- Insert the needle perpendicularly into the subcutaneous fat. Stabilize the syringe with two hands and have your thumb ready on the plunger to avoid the pain of needle wobble until the skin needle site is numb. Inject the first visible 0.5 ml bleb and then pause. Wait 15 to 45 seconds until the patient tells you that all needle pain is gone. Inject the rest of the 4 ml slowly (over 2 minutes) without moving the needle.

TIPS AND TRICKS FOR PERFORMING TRIGGER THUMB OR FINGER SURGERY WITH THE WIDE AWAKE APPROACH

- The patient needs to look at the fingers to get them to move, since he or she cannot feel the numbed digit. Although most patients don't mind looking at the wound, you can cover the wound with a towel as the patient flexes all fingers together while looking at them.

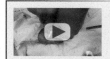

Clip 21-3 Trigger thumb surgery.

- Many patients are interested in looking at the tendon to understand the nature of their problem. Offer patients a guided tour of their trigger finger surgery. Many will accept and be delighted that they were given the opportunity to experience seeing the inside of their hand. You can put a mask on the patient, show him the tendon and have him watch it move. Many patients love this. Some patients have told others it is something they need to put on their bucket list!

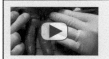

Clip 21-4 Wide awake trigger finger surgery

- Outside the operating room, inject two to four patients who will undergo relatively straightforward procedures such as trigger finger or thumb release, carpal tunnel release, and excision of a ganglion cyst outside the operating room before operating on the first patient. This gives at least half an hour for the local anesthetic to work both for lidocaine numbing and for epinephrine vasoconstriction. It takes 26 minutes to achieve peak vasoconstriction in humans after 1:100,000 epinephrine injection (level I evidence).[3]

- After you inject the first patient, most of them usually feel well enough to go sit in the waiting area for their surgery. You can then inject the second patient, then the third one. Next you can perform the surgery on the first patient. While the nurse turns over the room after the first one, you can inject the fourth patient.

We use Desmarres or vein retractors, which help to keep the fat out of the way and show the sheath.

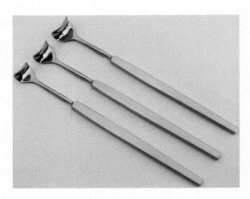

- Have your assistant push down on the Desmarres retractors to keep the fat out of the way and decrease the small amount of bleeding that sometimes occurs, especially if the patient is hypertensive or receiving anticoagulants.

- You can educate the patient during the local anesthetic injection (3 minutes) and during the surgery and bandage application (10 minutes). This gives you 13 minutes of patient education time, which will serve to decrease your complication rate and decrease the time you would spend educating the patient in the office (see Chapter 8).

References

1. Braithwaite BD, Robinson GJ, Burge PD. Haemostasis during carpal tunnel release under local anaesthesia: a controlled comparison of a tourniquet and adrenaline infiltration. J Hand Surg Br 18:184, 1993.
2. Ralte P, Selvan D, Morapudi S, Kumar G, Waseem M. Haemostasis in open carpal tunnel release: tourniquet vs local anaesthetic and adrenaline. Open Orthop J 4:234, 2010.
3. McKee DE, Lalonde DH, Thoma A, Glennie DL, Hayward JE. Optimal time delay between epinephrine injection and incision to minimize bleeding. Plast Reconstr Surg 131:811, 2013.

CHAPTER 22
DE QUERVAIN RELEASE

Donald H. Lalonde, Alistair Phillips

ADVANTAGES OF WALANT VERSUS SEDATION AND TOURNIQUET IN DE QUERVAIN RELEASE

- You can see active movement differentiating the abductor pollicis longus (APL) and the extensor pollicis brevis (EPB) so you can identify and release both compartments.

- A De Quervain release is such a short and simple operation that eliminating the tourniquet and sedation, with their associated discomforts and inconveniences, is good for both you and the patient.

- All of the general advantages listed in Chapter 2 apply to both the surgeon and the patient.

WHERE TO INJECT THE LOCAL ANESTHETIC FOR DE QUERVAIN RELEASE

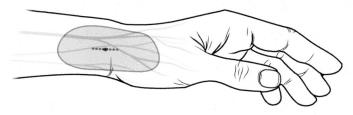

Inject 10 ml of 1% lidocaine with 1:100,000 epinephrine (buffered with 10 ml lido/epi:1 ml of 8.4% sodium bicarbonate) subcutaneously in the center of the incision area.

- See Chapter 1, Atlas, for more illustrations of the anatomy of diffusion of tumescent local anesthetic in the forearm, wrist, and hand.

SPECIFICS OF MINIMAL PAIN INJECTION OF LOCAL ANESTHETIC IN DE QUERVAIN RELEASE

- Inject just under the skin. There is no need to inject into the sheath; this would only add unnecessary pain. The local anesthetic will diffuse into the sheath if you wait half an hour.

- Since the skin on the radial wrist is thin and elastic, you can pinch it lightly and insert the needle into the pinched and elevated skin to add the sensory "noise" of pressure to decrease the pain from the first needle insertion. You can also move the skin into the needle tip. Ask the patient to look away.

- There is no need to move the needle from the initial placement site under the skin. The local anesthetic will go everywhere it needs to go. Think of it as an extravascular Bier block injected only where you need it.

- We inject the anesthetic solution a minimum of 30 minutes before surgery to allow the epinephrine to take optimal effect and provide an adequately dry working field, as outlined in Chapters 4 and 14.

- We inject supine patients lying down on stretchers in a waiting area to decrease the risk of their fainting (see Chapter 6).

- To minimize the pain of injection, inject with a fine 27-gauge needle (not a 25-gauge) into the red dot injection point at the center of the incision.

- Insert the first needle perpendicularly into the subcutaneous fat. Have your thumb ready on the plunger to avoid needle wobble pain until the skin needle site is numb. Inject the first visible 0.5 ml bleb and then pause. Ask the patient to tell you when the needle pain is all gone. When he or she says the pain is gone, inject the rest of the 10 ml slowly (over 2 to 3 minutes) without moving the needle.

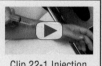

Clip 22-1 Injection and surgery for De Quervain synovitis. (Note that lignocaine is the same as lidocaine.)

TIPS AND TRICKS FOR PERFORMING DE QUERVAIN RELEASE WITH THE WIDE AWAKE APPROACH

- The patient may need to look at the thumb to get it to move, since it is partially numbed. Although most patients do not mind looking at the wound, you can cover the wound with a towel as the patient flexes and extends the thumb.

- Many patients are interested in looking at the tendon to understand the nature of their problem. You can put a mask on them, then show them the tendon and watch it move. Many patients love this. Some will tell others it is something they need to put on their bucket list!

- Desmarres or vein retractors help to keep the fat away and show the sheath (see Chapter 21).

- Field sterility is well suited to this brief operation to increase efficiency (see Chapters 10 and 14).

CHAPTER 23

DUPUYTREN'S CONTRACTURE

Duncan McGrouther, Jason Wong, Donald H. Lalonde

ADVANTAGES OF WALANT VERSUS SEDATION AND TOURNIQUET IN DUPUYTREN'S CONTRACTURE

- With the wide awake approach, you can see how much active extension the patient can really achieve after cord resection and before the skin is closed. You and the patient both find out during surgery whether or not the patient is likely to regain full active extension, thus avoiding the patient's having unrealistic expectations after surgery.

- Many of these patients are older and could have problems with general anesthesia and sedation because of medical comorbidities. With WALANT, they will just get up and go home as they do after they have a dental procedure.

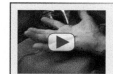

Clip 23-1 Verifying active extension with active movement after cord resection.

- Patients get to see that the cord and nodule are gone as they watch themselves moving their fingers through a full range of motion before the skin is closed. They realize that their fingers can work well once they get past the postoperative discomfort and stiffness.[1,2]

- Procedures requiring correction of multiple digits and revisions are not time limited by the use of a tourniquet.

- When a patient is being treated for recurrent Dupuytren's contracture, his or her mindset may be quite different than during a primary surgery for the condition. The patient may feel that during the initial repair there was minimal follow-up and perhaps not enough discussion about the fact that the disease would likely recur in the future. The wide awake procedure allows you to have a prolonged consultation with the patient during the surgery to discuss the recurrent nature of this condition and postoperative rehabilitation options.

- All of the general advantages listed in Chapter 2 apply to both the surgeon and the patient.

WHERE TO INJECT THE LOCAL ANESTHETIC FOR DUPUYTREN'S CONTRACTURE

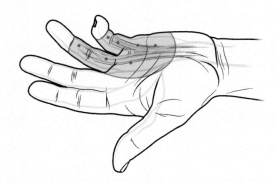

Inject up to 25 ml of 1% lidocaine with 1:100,000 epinephrine (buffered with 10 ml lido/epi:1 ml of 8.4% sodium bicarbonate).

- See Chapter 1, Atlas, for more illustrations of the anatomy of diffusion of tumescent local anesthetic in the forearm, wrist, and hand.

SPECIFICS OF MINIMALLY PAINFUL INJECTION OF LOCAL ANESTHETIC IN DUPUYTREN'S CONTRACTURE

- Inject supine patients lying down on stretchers before they come into the operating room, as outlined in Chapters 4, 5, and 14, to give the lidocaine and epinephrine time to work optimally and to decrease the risk of their fainting (see Chapter 6).

- To minimize the pain of injection, start with a fine 27-gauge needle (not a 25-gauge).

- Ask the patient to look away. Press with a fingertip just proximal to the injection site before you put in the needle to add the sensory "noise" of pressure to decrease the pain.

- Insert the needle perpendicularly into the subcutaneous fat in the most proximal point of the palm where you are likely to dissect. Stabilize the syringe with two hands and have your thumb ready on the plunger to avoid the pain of needle wobble until the skin needle site is numb. Inject the first visible 0.5 ml bleb and then pause. Wait 15 to 45 seconds until the patient tells you that all the needle pain is gone. Inject the rest of the first 10 ml slowly (over 2 to 3 minutes).

- Slowly advance the needle down below the fascia after putting the first 2 to 3 ml under the skin, and inject the last 7 ml there after aspirating to be sure the needle is not in a large vessel. It is ideal to wait 30 minutes while you do something else that is a good use of your time; this will allow full anesthesia of all of the distal nerves, and the epinephrine has time to vasoconstrict maximally.

- Inject another 9 ml in the distal palm (3 ml on either side of and between the two cords) now that the distal palm and digital nerves are numb.

- The cords can act as a barrier to the diffusion of local anesthetic. This is why you may need to inject on both sides of a cord. You should be able to see and palpate the local anesthetic under the skin at the site where you will make an incision and dissect.

- Inject another 2 ml in the middle of each proximal and middle phalanx wherever you are going to dissect. If you are going to dissect into the distal phalanx, you will only need 1 ml in the middle of the subcutaneous fat there.

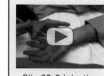

Clip 23-2 Injecting local anesthetic for Dupuytren's surgery.

- If you are going to be doing forceful joint manipulation or joint dissection, you may well need another 4 ml proximal to the dorsal MP joint as well as on the ulnar side of the small finger to make sure all dorsal joint branches are blocked.

TIPS AND TRICKS FOR PERFORMING DUPUYTREN'S CONTRACTURE SURGERY WITH THE WIDE AWAKE APPROACH

- Your first WALANT case should not be a Dupuytren's procedure. Secondary Dupuytren's surgeries are clearly even harder. This operation can be difficult for novice surgeons and trainees and can increase the risk of nerve damage. You should be comfortable with both WALANT and Dupuytren surgery before embarking on this procedure with the wide awake approach.

- WALANT surgery is not bloodless surgery. Dupuytren's, especially recurrent Dupuytren's, is the least dry operation in wide awake surgery. This is because the cords frequently wrap around the digital arteries, which are still pumping blood when bathed with 1:100,000 epinephrine. Their little branches bleed when avulsed by cord dissection. We recommend that you not perform Dupuytren's with WALANT until you are comfortable using WALANT for other procedures.

- One concern with performing Dupuytren's fasciectomy with this technique is that the blood in the field of view can obscure the disease. It is possible that you can leave disease behind that you might have removed under a bloodless field approach.

- You can apply a loose, uninflated tourniquet to the upper arm as a safety net.

- Patients need to look at the fingers to get them to move, since they cannot feel the numbed fingers. Although most patients do not mind looking at the wound, you can cover the wound with a towel as they flex all fingers together while looking at them.

- For dermofasciectomy, our preferred full-thickness skin graft donor site is the inner upper arm, 5 cm above the medial epicondyle and below the tourniquet (if you apply one). Clearly, this area will require further local anesthesia.

- Also for dermofasciectomy, we restrict the resection to the proximal segment of the digit, whereas Logan's group[3] has generally recommended extending further proximally. We remove a short segment of longitudinal cord at the distal palmar crease to release a contracted MP joint. However, we leave Dupuytren's tissues proximal and distal to the grafted area as, relieved from tension, they regress.

References

1. Denkler K. Dupuytren's fasciectomies in 60 consecutive digits using lidocaine with epinephrine and no tourniquet. Plast Reconstr Surg 115:802, 2005.
2. Nelson R, Higgins A, Conrad J, Bell M, Lalonde D. The wide-awake approach to Dupuytren's disease: fasciectomy under local anesthetic with epinephrine. Hand (N Y) 5:117, 2010.
3. Armstrong JR, Hurren JS, Logan AM. Dermofasciectomy in the management of Dupuytren's disease. J Bone Joint Surg Br 82:90, 2000.

CHAPTER 24
FLEXOR SHEATH GANGLION

Donald H. Lalonde

ADVANTAGES OF WALANT VERSUS SEDATION AND TOURNIQUET IN FLEXOR SHEATH GANGLION SURGERY

- Patients no longer have to go through all the inconveniences of sedation, a tourniquet, or general anesthesia for such a minor operation.
- All of the general advantages listed in Chapter 2 apply to both the surgeon and the patient.

WHERE TO INJECT THE LOCAL ANESTHETIC FOR FLEXOR SHEATH GANGLION SURGERY

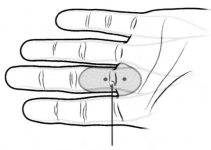

Inject 2 ml of 1% lidocaine with 1:100,000 epinephrine (buffered with 10 ml lido/epi: 1 ml of 8.4% sodium bicarbonate) in each of the two red injection points shown on the distal palm and proximal phalanx. First inject the palmar red dot injection point, then the proximal phalanx.

Flexor sheath ganglion

- See Chapter 1, Atlas, for more illustrations of the anatomy of diffusion of tumescent local anesthetic in the forearm, wrist, and hand.

SPECIFICS OF MINIMALLY PAINFUL INJECTION OF LOCAL ANESTHETIC IN FLEXOR SHEATH GANGLION SURGERY

- The palmar/digital crease ligaments create a natural barrier to diffusion of local anesthetic. This is why you need to inject on both sides of the crease.

- Inject in the fat just under the skin, aiming midway between the two digital nerves so you do not damage either one. There is no need to inject into the sheath; this would only add unnecessary pain. The local anesthetic will diffuse into the sheath during the waiting period.

- If you inject into the sheath, the local anesthetic will diffuse up the sheath into the whole finger or thumb. With enough pressure, the sheath will "explode" or burst. This will cause pain and send the epinephrine and lidocaine to the very end of the digit. This can cause a white fingertip. As with almost all white fingertips, it will eventually pink up. However, phentolamine can be injected to reverse the vasoconstriction (see Chapter 3).

- We inject the anesthetic solution a minimum of 30 minutes before surgery to allow the epinephrine to take optimal effect and provide an adequately dry working field, as outlined in Chapters 4 and 14.

- We inject supine patients lying down on stretchers in a waiting area before they come into the procedure room to decrease the risk of their fainting (see Chapter 6).

- To minimize the pain of injection, start with a 27-gauge needle (not a 25-gauge).

- Ask the patient to look away. Press with a fingertip just proximal to the injection site before you put in the needle to add the sensory "noise" of pressure to decrease the pain.

- First inject 2 ml in the palmar red dot injection point, then 2 ml in the proximal phalanx.

- Insert the needle perpendicularly into the subcutaneous fat. Stabilize the syringe with two hands and have your thumb ready on the plunger to avoid the pain of needle wobble until the skin needle site is numb. Inject the first visible 0.5 ml bleb and then pause. Wait 15 to 45 seconds until the patient tells you that all needle pain is gone. Inject the rest of the first 2 ml slowly (over 1 minute) without moving the needle. Then inject the proximal phalanx red dot injection point.

TIPS AND TRICKS FOR PERFORMING FLEXOR SHEATH GANGLION SURGERY WITH THE WIDE AWAKE APPROACH

- Desmarres or vein retractors help to keep the fat away and show the sheath with the ganglion.

- Field sterility is ideal for this brief operation and will increase efficiency (see Chapter 10).

CHAPTER 25
SMALL SOFT TISSUE OPERATIONS

Donald H. Lalonde, Jason Wong, Shu Guo Xing, Jin Bo Tang

ADVANTAGES OF WALANT VERSUS SEDATION AND TOURNIQUET IN SKIN CANCER EXCISION

- The large volume of tumescent local anesthetic used in this technique actually hydrodissects the tumor off the paratenon for you. This promotes the take of a skin graft and creates a nice tissue plane, permitting you to get under the cancer for complete excision of the tumor.

- Many of these patients are older and may have problems with general anesthesia and sedation because of medical comorbidities. With WALANT, they will simply get up and go home after the procedure, just like after they have a dental procedure.

- You can educate patients during surgery about how important it is that they keep their hand elevated and "on strike," doing absolutely nothing with it for the next week while the skin graft takes. At the end of the procedure, patients can sit up and elevate their hand with total understanding of what to do. If patients are sedated or undergo general anesthesia, they may not understand what to do and may be too groggy during postoperative recovery to grasp patient teaching. They may well keep their hand dependent and may even have problems with vomiting, which could lead to further hematoma under the graft. They may require hospital admission for the procedure to get safe general anesthesia and monitoring.

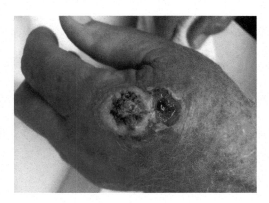

Squamous cell skin cancer in an 89-year-old man who was receiving anticoagulants.

- See Chapter 8 for a clip on giving a patient advice while excising skin cancer from the hand.

- All of the general advantages listed in Chapter 2 apply to both the surgeon and the patient.

WHERE TO INJECT THE LOCAL ANESTHETIC FOR SKIN CANCER EXCISION

In this patient we injected at least 20 ml of buffered 1% lidocaine with 1:100,000 epinephrine (buffered with 10 ml lido/epi:1 ml of 8.4% sodium bicarbonate). We injected from proximal to distal all around and under the tumor edge. We let the tumescent local anesthetic lift the tumor away from the tendons.

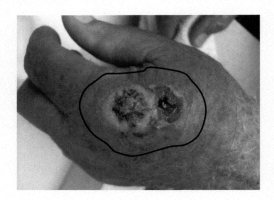

SPECIFICS OF MINIMALLY PAINFUL INJECTION OF LOCAL ANESTHETIC IN SKIN CANCER EXCISION

- We inject the anesthetic solution a minimum of 30 minutes before surgery to allow the epinephrine to take optimal effect and provide an adequately dry working field, as outlined in Chapters 4 and 14.

- We inject supine patients on stretchers in a waiting area outside the procedure room to decrease the risk of their fainting (see Chapter 6). We then operate on other patients while waiting for the epinephrine to work.

- To minimize the pain of injection, start with a fine 27-gauge needle (not a 25-gauge) into the most proximal injection point. This point is marked at least 1 cm proximal to the most proximal place you are likely to dissect.

- Ask the patient to look away. Press with a fingertip just proximal to the injection site before you put in the needle to add the sensory "noise" of pressure to decrease the pain.

- Insert the first needle perpendicularly into the subcutaneous fat. Stabilize the syringe with two hands to avoid needle wobble pain until the skin needle site is numb. Inject the first visible 0.5 ml bleb and then pause. Wait 15 to 45 seconds until the patient tells you that all needle pain is gone. Inject the rest of the first 10 ml slowly (over 2 minutes) without moving the needle.

- Reinsert the needle farther distally into skin that is within 1 cm of clearly vasoconstricted white skin that has functioning lidocaine and epinephrine so that needle reinsertion is pain free.

- Continue injecting from proximal to distal, blowing the local anesthetic slowly ahead of the needle so there is always at least 1 cm of visible or palpable local anesthetic ahead of the sharp needle tip that the patient would feel if you advanced it into "live" nerves. "Blow slow before you go." (See Chapter 5 for further tips on how to inject the local anesthetic with minimal pain.)

- Do not insert the needle in the tumor itself. Blow all around it first, from proximal to distal. You will elevate the tumor off the tendons with the large volume of tumescent local anesthetic.

- The more volume that you inject, the greater the loose tissue between the epitenon and the cancer will be elevated so that you will be able to retain epitenon and yet completely excise the cancer.

TIPS AND TRICKS FOR PERFORMING SKIN CANCER EXCISION WITH THE WIDE AWAKE APPROACH

- We performed a wide awake skin cancer excision in an 89-year-old man in a minor procedure room with field sterility (see Chapter 10).

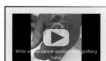

Clip 25-1 Surgical sequence and result in an 89-year-old patient.

- We waited for at least a half an hour between local anesthetic injection and excision of the tumor to allow the epinephrine to reach maximal vasoconstriction. We performed a couple of carpal tunnel releases on other patients after injecting this patient and while we were waiting for clotting after his cancer excision, so we used our time productively throughout.

- We marked the incision line before injecting the local anesthetic. The skin is healthy where it is soft and folds as you push it into the rigid cancer with your finger. The healthy skin becomes tumescent and no longer folds readily after you have injected the local anesthetic.

- We harvested a split-thickness skin graft with a 10 blade on the loose skin of the arm. We then excised the exposed dermis of the donor site and closed the wound primarily with buried dermal sutures. No suture removal was required. It healed nicely as a line scar much more quickly than it would have healed as a split-thickness donor site.

- After excising the skin cancer, we covered the wound with a saline-soaked gauze and wrapped it with a 3-inch Kling bandage. The patient (who was receiving anticoagulants) held it in elevation without moving his fingers. We waited another 45 minutes for the bleeding to stop completely, performing other small hand surgery cases while waiting. We removed the bandage and the clots over the epitenon and applied skin graft to most of the wound on the epitenon over the tendons. In this case, we used no cautery and tied off no veins, because we did not have to. We do have cautery in our minor procedure rooms but seldom use it, since the epinephrine vasoconstriction is usually adequate. We immobilized the hand with a volar splint for a week and reminded the patient that he should keep his hand "on strike," elevated without movement during the week. We got a full take of the graft we applied and a complete excision of the cancer.

TIPS AND TRICKS FOR PERFORMING LIPOMA EXCISION ON THE FOREARM WITH THE WIDE AWAKE APPROACH

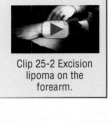

Clip 25-2 Excision lipoma on the forearm.

- We use the same injection technique as described above and in Chapters 4 and 5.

- If less than 50 ml is required, we use premixed 1% lidocaine with 1:100,000 epinephrine. If 50 to 100 ml is required, we dilute with saline solution to a concentration of 0.5% lidocaine with 1:200,000 epinephrine. If 100 to 200 ml is required, we dilute with saline solution to a concentration of 0.25% lidocaine with 1:400,000 epinephrine (all solutions buffered with 10 ml 1% lido/1:100,000 epi:1 ml of 8.4% sodium bicarbonate).

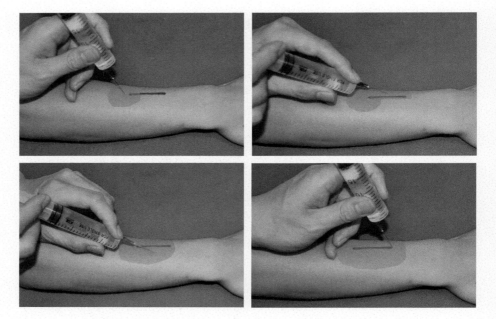

The goal of the injection is to get at least 1 cm of firm, white, tumesced skin and fat on either side of any incision or surrounding any dissection area. In this case, we used 20 ml of 1% lidocaine with 1:100,000 epinephrine buffered with 2 ml of 8.4% sodium bicarbonate.

CHAPTER 26

ARTHROPLASTY OF THE PROXIMAL INTERPHALANGEAL JOINT

Donald H. Lalonde

ADVANTAGES OF WALANT VERSUS SEDATION AND TOURNIQUET IN ARTHROPLASTY OF THE PROXIMAL INTERPHALANGEAL (PIP) JOINT

- If you choose a dorsal approach, you can see that you have repaired the extensor mechanism properly to get the best possible active extension without rupture of the repair. You watch the patient take the finger through a comfortable pain-free range of motion before skin closure. Sometimes the closing sutures in the extensor tendon will burst with intraoperative testing of full flexion and extension of the PIP joint. It is better to know that and fix it before you close the skin so that a boutonniere deformity does not develop later.

- Patients get to see that their previously stiff joint now moves as they watch themselves flexing their finger before the skin is closed. They realize that their hand will work well once they get past the postoperative discomfort and stiffness.

- Through intraoperative teaching and patients' ability to observe the repair, they will have a realistic expectation of the best possible outcome of range of movement when they leave the operating room.

- You are sure that the motion is optimal before closing the wound. You can adjust the tissues around the implant based on what you see with active movement.

- All of the general advantages listed in Chapter 2 apply to both the surgeon and the patient.

WHERE TO INJECT THE LOCAL ANESTHETIC FOR PIP JOINT ARTHROPLASTY

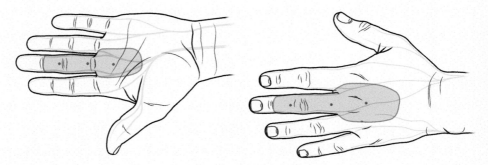

Palmar injections: Inject 4 ml of 1% lidocaine with 1:100,000 epinephrine (buffered with 10 ml lido/epi:1 ml of 8.4% sodium bicarbonate) in the most proximal red injection point on the palmar side. Do the most proximal dorsal injection next, and then inject 2 ml in the middle of the palmar proximal and middle phalanges in the subcutaneous fat. *Dorsal injections:* Inject 4 ml of 1% lidocaine with 1:100,000 epinephrine (buffered with 10 ml lido/epi:1 ml of 8.4% sodium bicarbonate) in the proximal red injection dot on the dorsal hand. Do the two palmar injections next, and then inject 2 ml in the middle of the dorsal proximal and middle phalanges in the subcutaneous fat.

- See Chapter 1, Atlas, for more illustrations of the anatomy of diffusion of tumescent local anesthetic in the forearm, wrist, and hand.

SPECIFICS OF MINIMALLY PAINFUL INJECTION OF LOCAL ANESTHETIC IN PIP JOINT ARTHROPLASTY

- Inject just under the skin. There is no need to inject into the sheath. It would only add unnecessary pain. The local anesthetic will diffuse into the sheath.

- Inject the anesthetic solution a minimum of 30 minutes before surgery to allow the epinephrine to take optimal effect and provide an adequately dry working field as outlined in Chapters 4 and 14.

- We inject supine patients lying down on stretchers to decrease the risk of their fainting (see Chapter 6).

- To minimize the pain of injection, start with a fine 27-gauge needle (not a 25-gauge).

- Ask the patient to look away. Press with a fingertip just proximal to the injection site before you put in the needle to add the sensory "noise" of pressure to decrease the pain.

- Insert the first needle perpendicularly into the subcutaneous fat. Stabilize the syringe with two hands to avoid the pain of needle wobble until the skin needle site is numb. Inject the first visible 0.5 ml bleb and then pause. Wait 15 to 45 seconds until the patient tells you that all the needle pain is gone. Inject the rest of the 4 ml slowly (over 1 to 2 minutes) without moving the needle.

- In this operation, inject 4 ml in the most proximal red dot injection point of the palm first, and then inject 4 ml in the most proximal red dot injection point of the dorsal hand right after that. This will give at least a little time for the distal injection points to numb up before you inject them.

- The distal injections are for the epinephrine vasoconstriction effect, since the skin is already numb from the proximal nerve blocks.

IF YOU ARE WORKING WITH AN ANESTHESIOLOGIST

- Ask him or her to use only propofol. Inject the lidocaine with epinephrine as soon as the propofol permits pain-free injection of local anesthetic. The anesthesiologist can then wake the patient right away while you are scrubbing, prepping, and draping so you can get the benefit of intraoperative patient teaching (Chapter 8) and fully cooperative pain-free movement. Suggest that the anesthesia provider avoid opiates and amnestics to prevent nausea and permit the patient to remember your intraoperative advice and discussions. This allows the patient to know what kind of result he or she can achieve with therapy.

TIPS AND TRICKS FOR PERFORMING PIP JOINT ARTHROPLASTY WITH THE WIDE AWAKE APPROACH

- We do not worry about minor bleeding from cut skin edges, because most little bleeders will stop spontaneously.

- After implant placement, get the patient to take the fingers through a full range of motion. You may want to make adjustments in the bone to improve the movement you see before you repair the soft tissues.

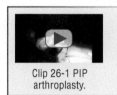

Clip 26-1 PIP arthroplasty.

- After soft tissue closure, ask the patient to take the fingers through a full range of motion. You may want to make adjustments in the extensor tendon closure to improve the movement you see before you let the patient leave the operating room.

- The patient needs to look at the fingers to get them to move, because he or she cannot feel the numbed finger. Although most patients do not mind looking at the wound, you can cover the wound with a towel as the patient flexes all fingers together while looking at them.

- Many patients are interested in looking at the opened finger to understand the nature of their problem. You can mask the patients and show them the tendons and joint. Have them watch their finger move. They will remember how well it works, and this will motivate them to achieve that same movement with therapy.

CHAPTER 27
TRAPEZIECTOMY WITH OR WITHOUT LIGAMENT RECONSTRUCTION FOR THUMB BASAL JOINT ARTHRITIS

Donald H. Lalonde, Peter C. Amadio, Geoff Cook

ADVANTAGES OF WALANT VERSUS SEDATION AND TOURNIQUET IN TRAPEZIECTOMY

- After you remove the trapezium, you can see whether the base of the metacarpal impinges on the scaphoid when you ask the patient to move the thumb all around. If it does, you can then add a ligament reconstruction in any way that you choose—with the abductor pollicis longus (APL), flexor carpi radialis (FCR), sutures, tightrope, and so on. After the suspension repair, you can verify that the reconstruction is keeping the metacarpal away from the scaphoid when you ask the patient to move the thumb again before you close the skin.

- Clip 27-1 discusses intraoperative decision-making about simple trapeziectomy versus a ligament reconstruction and tendon interposition (LRTI) based on what you see with active movement. (Also see the videos in the Tips and Tricks section of this chapter showing both impinging and nonimpinging metacarpals.)

Clip 27-1
Intraoperative decision-making about the appropriate procedure.

- After you finish with the basal joint work, you can assess the position and active movement of the thumb metacarpophalangeal (MP) joint. If the MP joint is still hyperextending, you can deal with it while the patient's hand is numbed. Ask the patient to move the thumb again after whichever MP joint surgery you choose. You can be sure both the basal and MP joints are actively moving well before you close the skin.

- Movement without impingement after the trapeziectomy may help you to decide to stop there and close the skin without ligament reconstruction.

- You can hear the thumb move through a full active range of motion after you remove the trapezium. You will sometimes hear remaining osteophytes grinding through the open wound with active movement. You can then find and remove them.

- Patients get to see that the thumb will be able to move through a full range of motion before the skin is closed. They know that all can work well once they get past the postoperative discomfort and stiffness.[1]

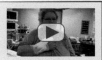

Clip 27-2 A patient
with medical
comorbidities
compares local and
general anesthesia.

- Many of these patients have medical comorbidities. Because they are not sedated in any way, they simply get up after surgery and go home, as they would after a dental procedure.

- All of the general advantages listed in Chapter 2 apply to both the surgeon and the patient.

WHERE TO INJECT THE LOCAL ANESTHETIC FOR A TRAPEZIECTOMY

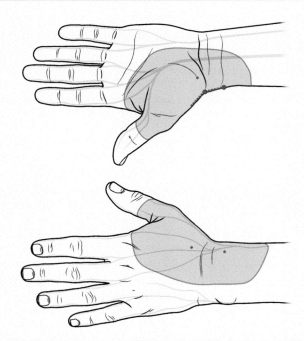

Inject a mixture of 40 ml of saline solution plus 40 ml of 1% lidocaine with 1:100,000 epinephrine (buffered with 10 ml lido/epi:1 ml of 8.4% sodium bicarbonate) plus 10 ml of 0.5% bupivacaine with 1:200,000 epinephrine.

- See Chapter 1, Atlas, for more illustrations of the anatomy of diffusion of tumescent local anesthetic in the forearm, wrist, and hand.

SPECIFICS OF MINIMALLY PAINFUL INJECTION OF LOCAL ANESTHETIC IN A TRAPEZIECTOMY

- Clip 27-4 shows real-time 8-minute injection of a patient with minimal pain for a trapeziectomy and ligament reconstruction. Surgery for this patient is shown in the ligament reconstruction in Clip 27-6, an APL procedure.

- Clip 27-5 shows cannula injection of local anesthetic for a trapeziectomy with a 40 mm long blunt-tipped 25-gauge cannula in a hole made with a 20-gauge needle (also see Chapter 5).

- We inject the anesthetic solution a minimum of 30 minutes before surgery to allow the epinephrine to take optimal effect and provide an adequately dry working field, as outlined in Chapters 3, 4, and 14.

- We inject supine patients lying down on stretchers in a waiting area to decrease the risk of their fainting (see Chapter 6).

- Start by injecting 10 ml of the mixture under the skin at the proximal trapeziectomy incision red dot injection point.

- After the first 10 ml, inject another 10 ml on the dorsal side of the trapezium, staying near the metacarpal base.

- After the second 10 ml on the dorsal side, inject another 10 ml on the volar side of the trapezium, staying near the metacarpal base.

- After the third 10 ml on the volar side, inject a fourth 10 ml slowly between the thumb and index metacarpal bases going from the dorsal articulation to the volar side where the metacarpals meet the trapezium, staying near the bone.

- Finally, distract (pull on) the thumb and inject 5 ml into the basal metacarpal trapezial joint. This last 5 ml can also be injected into the joint capsule under direct vision after the skin incision during the surgery.

- If performing an LRTI with the flexor carpi radialis, inject 20 to 40 ml of the mixture from proximal to distal so there is at least 2 cm of visible or palpable local anesthetic beyond everywhere you will dissect.

- If performing an LRTI with the abductor pollicis longus, you may need another 10 ml of the mixture over the proximal APL so there is at least 2 cm of visible or palpable local anesthetic outside of everywhere you will dissect. In Clip 27-6, an APL reconstruction, no further local anesthetic was needed after the original 40 ml.

- To minimize pain of injection, start with a fine 27-gauge needle (not a 25-gauge).

- Ask the patient to look away. Press with a fingertip just proximal to the injection site before you put in the needle to add the sensory "noise" of pressure to decrease the pain.

- Insert the first needle perpendicularly into the subcutaneous fat. Stabilize the syringe with two hands to avoid the pain of needle wobble until the skin needle site is numb. Inject the first visible 0.5 ml bleb and then pause. Wait 15 to 45 seconds until the patient tells you that all

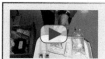

Clip 27-3 Mixing the local anesthetic solution for a trapeziectomy.

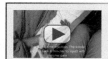

Clip 27-4 Real-time 8-minute injection of a patient.

Clip 27-5 Cannula injection of local anesthetic for a trapeziectomy.

the needle pain is gone. Inject the rest of the first 10 ml slowly (over 2 minutes) without moving the needle.

- When you have to reinsert the needle, always put it back into skin that is clearly white with epinephrine. If you reinsert within 1 cm of clearly white vasoconstricted skin that has functioning lidocaine and epinephrine, needle reinsertion will be pain free.

- Continue injecting from proximal to distal, blowing the local anesthetic slowly ahead of the needle so there is always at least 1 cm of visible or palpable local anesthesia ahead of the sharp needle tip point that the patient would feel if you advanced it into "live" nerves. "Blow slow before you go." (See Chapter 5 for further tips on how to inject local anesthetic with minimal pain.)

- The goal of the injection is to bathe local anesthetic 2 cm beyond wherever you think you even have a small chance of dissecting or inserting a K-wire.

- We keep the total dose of infiltration less than 7 mg/kg. If we need less than 50 ml of tumescent local anesthetic (see Chapter 4), we use premixed 1% lidocaine with 1:100,000 epinephrine (buffered with 10 ml lido/epi:1 ml of 8.4% sodium bicarbonate). If we need 50 to 100 ml, we dilute the 50 ml of 1% lidocaine with 1:100,000 epinephrine with 50 ml of saline solution to a concentration of 0.5% lidocaine with 1:200,000 epinephrine. If we need 100 to 200 ml of volume, we dilute 50 ml of 1% lidocaine with 1:100,000 epinephrine with 150 ml of saline solution to get 200 ml of 0.25% lidocaine with 1:400,000 epinephrine, which is clinically very effective.

IF YOU ARE WORKING WITH AN ANESTHESIOLOGIST

- Ask him or her to use only propofol. Inject the lidocaine with epinephrine as soon as the propofol permits pain-free injection of local anesthetic. The anesthesiologist can then wake the patient right away while you are scrubbing, prepping, and draping so you can get the benefit of intraoperative patient teaching (Chapter 8) and fully cooperative pain-free movement. Suggest that the anesthesia provider avoid administering opiates and amnestics to prevent nausea and permit the patient to remember your intraoperative advice and discussions.

TIPS AND TRICKS FOR PERFORMING A TRAPEZIECTOMY WITH THE WIDE AWAKE APPROACH

- Patients must look at the thumb to get it to move, because they cannot feel the numbed thumb. Although most patients don't mind looking at the wound, you can cover the wound with a towel as they move the thumb if they do mind looking at it.

- If you see the thumb metacarpal impinging on the scaphoid, you can perform a ligament reconstruction, as in Clip 27-6.

- In Clip 27-6, when the patient actively moved the thumb, this revealed metacarpal grinding on the scaphoid, so we decided to perform a Weilby suspension with half of the abductor pollicis longus.

- If the thumb metacarpal is not impinging on the scaphoid, you can stop at the trapeziectomy if you wish to, as in Clip 27-7.

- Many patients are interested in looking at the joint to understand the nature of their problem. You can mask the patient and show him or her the joint and watch it move. Many patients love this. Some patients will tell others it is something they need to put on their bucket list!

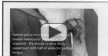

Clip 27-6 Ligament reconstruction with APL.

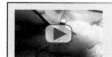

Clip 27-7 Watching the metacarpal move without grinding on scaphoid.

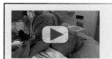

Clip 27-8 Patient impressions during trapeziectomy.

Reference

1. Farhangkhoee H, Lalonde J, Lalonde DH. Wide-awake trapeziectomy: video detailing local anesthetic injection and surgery. Hand 6:466, 2011.

CHAPTER 28

THUMB METACARPOPHALANGEAL JOINT FUSION AND ULNAR COLLATERAL LIGAMENT REPAIR

Donald H. Lalonde

ADVANTAGES OF WALANT VERSUS SEDATION AND TOURNIQUET IN THUMB METACARPOPHALANGEAL JOINT FUSION

- You can walk around the operating table and assess how the thumb looks with patient active movement after you fix the metacarpophalangeal (MCP) joint with K-wires. You and the patient can compare the active movement of the K-wired thumb to the normal thumb on the other hand.

- Patients can see the thumb position and their thumb move after you place the first K-wires. They can participate in choosing the final angle of fixation, because you can reposition the K-wires if you choose to do so.

- Both you and the patient leave the operating room with realistic expectations of final possible thumb movement.

- Patients get to see that the thumb will still be able to move before the skin is closed. They know that all can work well once they get past the postoperative discomfort and stiffness. They will be motivated to regain the movement they saw in the operating room.

- All of the general advantages listed in Chapter 2 apply to both the surgeon and the patient.

ADVANTAGES OF WALANT VERSUS SEDATION AND TOURNIQUET IN ULNAR COLLATERAL LIGAMENT REPAIR

- You can check the stability of the reconstructed MCP joint by observing active movement during the surgery.

- All of the other advantages listed above with fusion also apply.

WHERE TO INJECT THE LOCAL ANESTHETIC FOR THUMB MCP JOINT FUSION AND ULNAR COLLATERAL LIGAMENT REPAIR

Injection of the hand for thumb MP joint fusion and ulnar collateral ligament (UCL) repair. *Volar injection:* Inject 12 ml of 1% lidocaine with 1:100,000 epinephrine (buffered with 10 ml lido/epi:1 ml of 8.4% sodium bicarbonate). *Dorsal injection:* Inject 12 ml of 1% lidocaine with 1:100,000 epinephrine (buffered with 10 ml lido/epi:1 ml of 8.4% sodium bicarbonate).

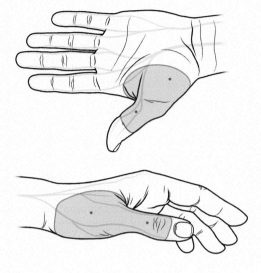

- See Chapter 1, Atlas, for more illustrations of the anatomy of diffusion of tumescent local anesthetic in the forearm, wrist, and hand.

SPECIFICS OF MINIMALLY PAINFUL INJECTION OF LOCAL ANESTHETIC IN THESE OPERATIONS

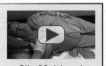

Clip 28-1 Local anesthetic injection for thumb MCP fusion or UCL repair.

- Clip 28-1 shows injection of local anesthetic for thumb MCP fusion or UCL repair. (See the surgery for this patient in Clip 28-2.)

- Inject 10 ml of the mixture under the skin on each of the volar and dorsal sides of the middle of the thumb metacarpal. Then inject 2 ml under the skin on each of the volar and dorsal sides of the middle of the thumb proximal phalanx.

- We inject the anesthetic solution a minimum of 30 minutes before surgery to allow the epinephrine to take optimal effect and provide an adequately dry working field as outlined in Chapters 4 and 14.

- We inject supine patients lying down on stretchers in a waiting area before they come into the operating room to decrease the risk of their fainting (see Chapter 6).

- To minimize the pain of injection (see Chapter 5), start with a 27-gauge needle (not a 25-gauge).

- Ask the patient to look away. Press with a fingertip just proximal to the injection site before you put in the needle to add the sensory "noise" of pressure to decrease the pain.

- Insert the first needle perpendicularly into the subcutaneous fat. Stabilize the syringe with two hands and have the thumb ready on the plunger to avoid needle wobble pain until the skin needle site is numb. Inject the first visible 0.5 cc bleb and then pause. Wait 15 to 45 seconds until the patient tells you that all the needle pain is gone. Inject the rest of the first 10 ml slowly (over 2 to 3 minutes) without moving the needle.

- In this operation, inject the first 10 ml in the most proximal part of the palmar thumb first, and then inject the next 10 ml in the most proximal part of the dorsal thumb right after that. Follow with the distal injections on the palmar and dorsal proximal phalanx, which are for the epinephrine vasoconstriction effect.

IF YOU ARE WORKING WITH AN ANESTHESIOLOGIST

- Ask him or her to use only propofol. Inject the lidocaine with epinephrine as soon as the propofol permits pain-free injection of local anesthetic. The anesthesiologist can then wake the patient right away while you are scrubbing, prepping, and draping so you can get the benefit of intraoperative patient teaching (Chapter 8) and fully cooperative pain-free movement. Suggest that the anesthesia provider avoid administering opiates and amnestics to prevent nausea and permit the patient to remember your intraoperative advice and discussions.

TIPS AND TRICKS FOR PERFORMING THESE OPERATIONS WITH THE WIDE AWAKE APPROACH

- Have the patient look at the thumb to verify that he or she feels the position is good and that the thumb is straight after inserting temporary K-wires. If you or the patient does not like the position after watching the thumb move, simply remove and replace the K-wires after adjusting the fusion position.

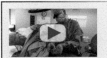

Clip 28-2 Thumb MCP fusion in the same patient in Clip 28-1.

- Have the patient move the other thumb and compare the two thumbs moving.

- Patients need to look at their thumb to get it to move, since they cannot feel the numbed thumb. Although most patients do not mind looking at the wound, you can cover the wound with a towel as they move the thumb if this seems appropriate.

- Consider performing this operation standing instead of sitting so you can easily walk around the table and ensure that the fused or reconstructed thumb looks good flexing and extending from all positions.

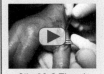

Clip 28-3 Thumb UCL repair.

CHAPTER 29
PROXIMAL INTERPHALANGEAL JOINT FUSION

Donald H. Lalonde

ADVANTAGES OF WALANT VERSUS SEDATION AND TOURNIQUET IN PROXIMAL INTERPHALANGEAL (PIP) JOINT FUSION

- Patients can help you select the angle of PIP fusion during the surgery. You insert temporary K-wires and let them look at and move the fingers of the hand. They may ask you for a little more flexion or extension.

- Patients get to see how much movement they will have once they get past the postoperative discomfort and stiffness.

- Patients leave the operating room with realistic expectations of their final ability to move. They are motivated to work with the therapists to regain what they have seen moving at surgery.

- All of the general advantages listed in Chapter 2 apply to both the surgeon and the patient.

WHERE TO INJECT THE LOCAL ANESTHETIC FOR PIP JOINT FUSION

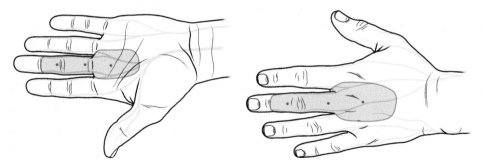

Palmar injections: Inject 4 ml of 1% lidocaine with 1:100,000 epinephrine (buffered with 10 ml lido/epi:1 ml of 8.4% sodium bicarbonate) in the most proximal red injection point on the palmar side. Perform the most proximal dorsal injection next, and then inject 2 ml in the subcutaneous fat in the middle of each of the palmar proximal and middle phalanges. *Dorsal injections:* Inject 4 ml of 1% lidocaine with 1:100,000 epinephrine (buffered with 10 ml lido/epi:1 ml of 8.4% sodium bicarbonate) in the proximal red injection dot on the dorsal hand. Perform the two palmar injections next, and then inject 2 ml in the subcutaneous fat in the middle of each of the dorsal proximal and middle phalanges.

- See Chapter 1, Atlas, for more illustrations of the anatomy of diffusion of tumescent local anesthetic in the forearm, wrist, and hand.

SPECIFICS OF MINIMALLY PAINFUL INJECTION OF LOCAL ANESTHETIC IN PIP JOINT FUSION

- Inject just under the skin. There is no need to inject into the sheath; this would only add unnecessary pain. The local anesthetic will diffuse into the sheath.

- Inject the anesthetic solution a minimum of 30 minutes before surgery to allow the epinephrine to take optimal effect and provide an adequately dry working field, as outlined in Chapters 4 and 14.

- We inject supine patients lying down on a stretcher in a waiting area before they come into the operating room, as outlined in Chapter 6, to decrease the risk of their fainting.

- To minimize the pain of injection, start with a fine 27-gauge needle (not a 25-gauge).

- Ask the patient to look away. Press with a fingertip just proximal to the injection site before you put in the needle to add the sensory "noise" of pressure to decrease the pain.

- Insert the first needle perpendicularly into the subcutaneous fat. Stabilize the syringe with two hands and have your thumb ready on the plunger to avoid the pain of needle wobble until the skin needle site is numb. Inject the first visible 0.5 ml bleb and then pause. Wait 15 to 45 seconds until the patient tells you that all the needle pain is gone. Inject the rest of the 4 ml slowly (over 2 minutes) without moving the needle.

- In this operation, inject the 4 ml in the most proximal part of the palm first, and then inject 4 ml in the most proximal part of the dorsal hand right after that. This will provide a little more time for the distal injection points in the phalanges to numb up before you inject them.

- The distal injections are for the epinephrine vasoconstriction effect, since the skin is already numb from the proximal nerve blocks.

IF YOU ARE WORKING WITH AN ANESTHESIOLOGIST

- Ask him or her to use only propofol. Inject the lidocaine with epinephrine as soon as the propofol permits pain-free injection of local anesthetic. The anesthesiologist can then wake the patient up right away while you are scrubbing, prepping, and draping so you can get the benefit of intraoperative patient teaching (Chapter 8) and fully cooperative pain-free movement. Suggest that the anesthesia provider avoid administering opiates and amnestics to prevent nausea and permit the patient to remember your intraoperative advice and discussions.

TIPS AND TRICKS FOR PERFORMING PIP JOINT FUSION WITH THE WIDE AWAKE APPROACH

- We do not worry about minor bleeding from cut skin edges, because most little bleeders will stop spontaneously.

- After temporary K-wire stabilization, have the patient test his or her active range of motion before final fusion. This will let you and the patient see that this is the best movement that he or she can achieve with the PIP joint in this position. (See the video of thumb MP joint fusion in Chapter 28, which illustrates this point.)

- Patients need to look at their fingers to get them to move, since they cannot feel the numbed finger. Although most patients do not mind looking at the wound, you can cover it with a gauze as they flex all the fingers together while looking at them.

- If you have patients participate in selecting the final angle of fusion, they may be more likely to be satisfied with the result. You can ask for their opinion after inserting temporary K-wires and having them see their resulting movement.

- Consider performing this operation standing so you can easily walk around the table and ensure that the fused finger looks good flexing and extending from all positions.

CHAPTER 30

WRIST ARTHROSCOPY

Elisabet Hagert, Donald H. Lalonde

ADVANTAGES OF WALANT VERSUS SEDATION AND TOURNIQUET IN WRIST ARTHROSCOPY

• Watching an awake patient move the wrist during WALANT wrist arthroscopy provides information not available from MRIs or from a sedated patient. It can be more useful as both a diagnostic and a therapeutic tool.

• Intraoperative active motion of the wrist can give you better information about the degree of ligament injury in situations such as a scapholunate or lunotriquetral injury. A cooperative, pain-free patient provides an "active" Geissler evaluation.[1]

• By performing dry or wet wrist arthroscopy using WALANT, patients can participate in the diagnosis and decision-making. This enhances their ability to take an active part in their treatment.

• You do not infuse water into the joint in dry wrist arthroscopy. This has advantages that make it valuable in diagnostic arthroscopy.[2] WALANT works well for this technique. The advantage with WALANT in dry arthroscopy is that detailed imaging of the wrist may be obtained to both diagnose and educate the patient during surgery.

• All of the general advantages listed in Chapter 2 apply to both the surgeon and the patient.

WHERE TO INJECT THE LOCAL ANESTHETIC FOR WRIST ARTHROSCOPY

Inject at least 20 to 30 ml of 1% lidocaine with 1:100,000 (available in North America) or 1:200,000 (available in Sweden) epinephrine (buffered with 10 ml lido/epi:1 ml of 8.4% sodium bicarbonate). Note that the higher concentration of epinephrine will increase the hemostatic effect and prolong the duration of anesthesia (see Chapter 4).

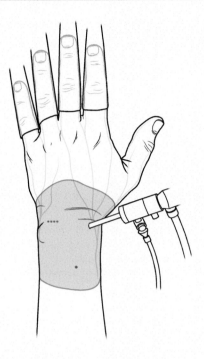

- See Chapter 1, Atlas, for more illustrations of the anatomy of diffusion of tumescent local anesthetic in the forearm, wrist, and hand.

SPECIFICS OF MINIMAL PAIN INJECTION OF LOCAL ANESTHETIC IN WRIST ARTHROSCOPY

- It is important to block the nerve branches innervating the dorsal wrist capsule so you can access pain-free portals.
- We inject patients lying down on stretchers in a waiting area before they come into the operating room to decrease the risk of their fainting (see Chapter 6).
- Slowly infiltrate at least 20 to 30 ml of buffered lidocaine with epinephrine to the dorsal aspect of the wrist to block the sensory branches of the radial, ulnar, and posterior interosseous nerves.[1] The infiltration should cover the area from the level of Lister's tubercle to the carpometacarpal joints.
- The goal of the injection is to bathe local anesthetic 2 cm beyond wherever you think you have even a small chance of dissecting in the wrist or forearm.

- To minimize the pain of injection, start with a 27-gauge needle (not a 25-gauge) in the most proximal red dot injection point.

- Ask the patient to look away. Press with a fingertip just proximal to the injection site before you put in the needle to add the sensory "noise" of pressure to decrease the pain.

- Insert the first needle perpendicularly into the subcutaneous fat. Stabilize the syringe with two hands and have your thumb ready on the plunger to avoid the pain of needle wobble until the skin needle site is numb. Inject the first visible 0.5 ml bleb and then pause. Wait 15 to 45 seconds until the patient tells you that all the needle pain is gone. Inject the rest of the first 10 ml slowly (over 2 minutes) without moving the needle.

- Reinsert the needle farther distally into skin that is within 1 cm of clearly vasoconstricted white skin that has functioning lidocaine and epinephrine so that needle reinsertion is pain free.

- Continue injecting from proximal to distal, blowing the local anesthetic slowly ahead of the needle so there is always at least 1 cm of visible or palpable local anesthetic ahead of the sharp needle tip that the patient would feel if you advanced it into "live" nerves. "Blow slow before you go." (See Chapter 5 for further tips on how to inject local anesthetic with minimal pain.)

- Following the subcutaneous infiltration, inject at least 2 ml of lidocaine-epinephrine into the radiocarpal joint to ensure anesthesia of the volar wrist capsule if shaving manipulation of the joint proves necessary.

- A technique using portal site anesthesia alone has been described, in which each portal is marked and injected with an average of 5 to 6 ml of local anesthetic.[3] Blocking the entire dorsal aspect of the wrist ensures a pain-free procedure and retains the option to convert from arthroscopic to open surgery with good anesthesia and hemostasis.

- We seldom use volar wrist portals. If you plan to use these, you must infiltrate subcutaneous volar anesthetic as well.[4]

- If you are going to manipulate the palmar structures as well, you should inject an additional 10 ml under the forearm fascia between the median and ulnar nerves on the palmar side 1 cm proximal to the wrist crease.

TIPS AND TRICKS FOR PERFORMING WRIST ARTHROSCOPY WITH THE WIDE AWAKE APPROACH

- Patients will still have sensation in their fingers. We recommend plastic finger traps for wrist traction, because the metal traps may be uncomfortable.

- Finger traction is not painful in itself; however, the patient will feel as though the fingers are cold and a little numb toward the end of the surgery. This will resolve as soon as the finger traps are removed.

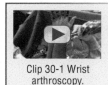

Clip 30-1 Wrist arthroscopy.

- When arthroscopic shaving is done, the patient will feel the vibrations but not feel pain. Explain this to your patient before you start shaving to reduce the patient's stress that may be caused by the sensation of vibrations.

IF YOU ARE WORKING WITH AN ANESTHESIOLOGIST

- Ask him or her to use only propofol. Inject the lidocaine with epinephrine as soon as the propofol permits pain-free injection of local anesthetic. The anesthesiologist can then wake the patient right away while you are scrubbing, prepping, and draping so you can get the benefit of intraoperative patient teaching (see Chapter 8) and fully cooperative pain-free movement. This will give the epinephrine a little time to become more effective. Suggest that the anesthesia provider avoid administering opiates and amnestics to prevent nausea and permit the patient to remember your intraoperative advice and discussions.

References

1. Hagert E, Lalonde D. Wide-awake wrist arthroscopy and open TFCC Repair. J Wrist Surg 1:55, 2012.
2. del Pinal F. Dry arthroscopy and its applications. Hand Clin 27:335, 2011.
3. Ong MT, Ho PC, Wong CW, Cheng SH, Tse WL. Wrist arthroscopy under portal site local anesthesia (PSLA) without tourniquet. J Wrist Surg 1:149, 2012.
4. Slutsky DJ, Nagle DJ. Wrist arthroscopy: current concepts. J Hand Surg Am 33:1228, 2008.

Chapter 31

Open Triangular Fibrocartilage Complex Repair

Elisabet Hagert, Donald H. Lalonde

ADVANTAGES OF WALANT VERSUS SEDATION AND TOURNIQUET IN OPEN TRIANGULAR FIBROCARTILAGE COMPLEX (TFCC) REPAIR

- A diagnostic wrist arthroscopy (see Chapter 30) often precedes this surgery to verify the need to perform a TFCC repair as a result of foveal detachment of the dorsal and/or volar radioulnar ligaments (DRUL/VRUL).

- Because the patient is awake, you can discuss the need to continue with an open repair. Thus the unsedated patient can actively participate in this decision.

- When performing the reattachment of the DRUL/VRUL to the fovea with either osteosutures or a bone anchor, you can test the tension in the ligaments with the patient's active movement.

- If you reattach the ligaments too loosely, you will see instability with the distal radioulnar joint (DRUJ) shift test.

- If you reattach the ligaments too tightly, the patient will not have full range of active pronation and supination.

- Because awake patients can see their hand move through a full range of pronation and supination after the reconstruction, they know that they can achieve it again after they go through postoperative immobilization and subsequent rehabilitation.

- All of the general advantages listed in Chapter 2 apply to both the surgeon and the patient.

WHERE TO INJECT THE LOCAL ANESTHETIC FOR OPEN TFCC REPAIR

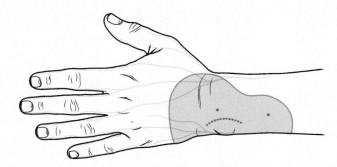

Inject 40 ml of 1% lidocaine with 1:100,000 (available in North America) or 1:200,000 (available in Sweden) (buffered with 10 ml lido/epi:1 ml of 8.4% sodium bicarbonate).

- See Chapter 1, Atlas, for more illustrations of the anatomy of diffusion of tumescent local anesthetic in the forearm, wrist, and hand.

SPECIFICS OF MINIMALLY PAINFUL INJECTION OF LOCAL ANESTHESIA IN OPEN TFCC REPAIR

- Inject the anesthetic solution a minimum of 30 minutes before surgery to allow the epinephrine to take optimal effect and provide an adequately dry working field, as outlined in Chapters 4 and 14.
- We inject supine patients lying down on stretchers in a waiting area to decrease the risk of their fainting (see Chapter 6).
- The tumescent local anesthetic will block the dorsal cutaneous branch of the ulnar nerve and the terminal branch of the posterior interosseous nerve to ensure a pain-free procedure.[1]
- Begin the injection 5 to 7 cm proximal to the DRUJ, along the ulnar border of the forearm. Slowly inject 20 ml along the ulnar border and dorsal distal ulna. Inject about 10 ml along the dorsal wrist, making sure to add 2 ml in the area of the PIN at the level of Lister's tubercle. Finally, inject the remaining 5 to 10 ml in the ulnocarpal region, with a few milliliters into the ulnocarpal joint for maximum effect.
- The goal of the injection is to bathe local anesthetic 2 cm beyond wherever you think you have even a small chance of dissecting.
- To minimize the pain of injection, use a 27-gauge needle (not a 25-gauge).

- Ask the patient to look away. Press with a fingertip just proximal to the injection site before you put in the needle to add the sensory "noise" of pressure to decrease the pain.

- Insert the first needle perpendicularly into the subcutaneous fat. Stabilize the syringe with two hands and have your thumb ready on the plunger to avoid the pain of needle wobble until the skin needle site is numb. Inject the first visible 0.5 ml bleb and then pause. Wait 15 to 45 seconds until the patient tells you that all the needle pain is gone. Inject the rest of the first 10 ml slowly (over 2 to 3 minutes) without moving the needle.

- Reinsert the needle farther distally within 1 cm of clearly vasoconstricted blanched skin that has functioning lidocaine and epinephrine so the needle reinsertion is pain free.

- Continue injecting from proximal to distal, blowing the local anesthesia slowly ahead of the needle so there is always at least 1 cm of visible or palpable local anesthetic ahead of the sharp needle tip that the patient would feel if you advanced it into "live" nerves. "Blow slow before you go." (See Chapter 5 for further tips on how to inject the local anesthesia with minimal pain.)

- We keep the total dose of infiltrated anesthetic to less than 7 mg/kg. If less than 50 ml will be required to produce tumescent local anesthesia, we use premixed 1% lidocaine with 1:100,000 epinephrine. If 50 to 100 ml is required, we dilute 50 ml of lidocaine and epinephrine with 50 ml of saline solution to a concentration of 0.5% lidocaine with 1:200,000 epinephrine.

- If you have access to blunt-tipped injection cannulas,[2] you can inject the local anesthetic more quickly than you can with a sharp needle tip in a minimally painful fashion (see Chapter 5).

IF YOU ARE WORKING WITH AN ANESTHESIOLOGIST

- Ask him or her to use only propofol. Inject the lidocaine with epinephrine as soon as the propofol permits pain-free injection of local anesthetic. The anesthesiologist can then wake the patient right away while you are scrubbing, prepping, and draping so you can get the benefit of intraoperative patient teaching (Chapter 8) and fully cooperative pain-free movement.

- This will give the epinephrine a little time to become more effective. Suggest that the anesthesia provider avoid administering opiates and amnestics to prevent nausea and permit patients to remember your intraoperative advice. Patients will also remember the range of motion they can achieve.

TIPS AND TRICKS FOR PERFORMING OPEN TFCC REPAIR WITH THE WIDE AWAKE APPROACH

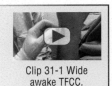

Clip 31-1 Wide awake TFCC.

- Make sure to use enough volume of local anesthetic to keep the patient pain free during surgery. Too much local anesthetic is always better than not enough—if you stay within a safe dosage range.

- Patients will still have sensation in their fingers unless you block the median and ulnar nerves on the volar aspect of the hand. You may want to use plastic finger traps for wrist traction, because metal traps may be uncomfortable.

- Finger traction is not painful in itself; however, the patient will feel as though the fingers are cold and a little numb toward the end of the surgery. This will resolve as soon as the finger traps are removed.

- When you drill the canals for the osteosutures or the bone anchor, the patient will feel the vibration in the distal ulna, but no pain. Explain this to the patient before you start drilling to reduce the stress that may be caused by the sensation of vibrations.

References

1. Hagert E, Lalonde D. Wide-awake wrist arthroscopy and open TFCC repair. J Wrist Surg 1:55, 2012.
2. Lalonde D, Wong A. Local anesthetics: what's new in minimal pain injection and best evidence in pain control. Plast Reconstr Surg 134(4 Suppl 2):40S, 2014.

CHAPTER 32

FLEXOR TENDON REPAIR OF THE FINGER

Jin Bo Tang, Shu Guo Xing, Jason Wong, Jeffrey Yao,
Donald H. Lalonde

ADVANTAGES OF WALANT VERSUS SEDATION AND TOURNIQUET IN FLEXOR TENDON REPAIR OF THE FINGER

INTRAOPERATIVE TESTING OF A REPAIR

- Intraoperative testing of a repair with WALANT (such as asking the patient to actively extend and flex the operated finger fully) can reveal gapping of a weak repair and decrease rupture rates.

- If you see the repair gapping after you ask the patient to make a full fist and completely straighten the fingers, you can repair the gap with more sutures, retest the repair to confirm that it is reliable with intraoperative flexion testing, and then close the skin. This is like testing blood flow through a microvascular anastomosis to avoid failure.

- You are less likely to have to perform a secondary surgery for rupture repair if you test the repair intraoperatively by having the patient take the fingers through a full range of flexion and extension before skin closure.[1,2]

- Clip 32-2 contains other useful tips on avoiding rupture during and after surgery.

Clip 32-1 How WALANT has improved flexor tendon repair results.

WALANT CAN DECREASE TENOLYSIS RATES

- You are less likely to have to come back for tenolysis if you see the patient take the fingers through a full range of motion before you close the skin. You know the repair will fit through the pulleys. You only need to vent (divide) the parts of the pulleys that are required to obtain a full range of intraoperative active movement of the finger, including all of A4 or one half to two thirds of the distal A2 pulley. (See Clip 32-12 of A4 pulley venting with no bowstringing in the Tips and Tricks section of this chapter.)

- Seeing the patient make a full fist and completely straighten out the fingers without gapping at surgery gives the surgeon full confidence to allow up to half a fist of true active movement 3 to 5 days later.

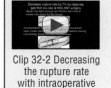

Clip 32-2 Decreasing the rupture rate with intraoperative testing.

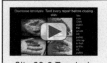

Clip 32-3 Tenolysis rate decreased by ensuring the repair fits through all pulleys.

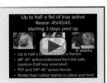

Clip 32-4 Half a fist of true active movement.

- We have abandoned the use of Kleinert rubber bands as well as "place-and-hold" active extension and passive flexion in favor of true active movement in our postoperative regimen. We feel that up to half a fist of true active finger flexion and full finger phalangeal joint extension has improved the results of our repair. We allow full wrist extension, up to half a fist of active flexion (45 degrees of active metacarpophalangeal [MP] extension, and up to 45 degrees of active proximal interphalangeal [PIP] and distal interphalangeal [DIP] flexion). Half a fist of flexion translates to 1 cm of active flexor digitorum profundus (FDP) tendon glide. (See Clip 32-16 on 1 cm of tendon glide with half a fist in the Tips and Tricks section of this chapter.)

INTRAOPERATIVE PATIENT EDUCATION

- The ability to educate the patient intraoperatively during a WALANT flexor tendon repair decreases rupture and tenolysis rates because the patient sees it all and remembers the consequences of moving versus using the hand after surgery.

- WALANT allows you and the hand therapist (see Chapter 15) to assess patients and educate them for up to 60 uninterrupted minutes during the surgery. We think this has been very important in improving our results.

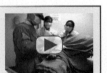

Clip 32-5 Intraoperative patient education decreases rupture and tenolysis rates.

- You are able to talk to unsedated patients, who usually become very interested in learning about the procedure during the operation. Patients have the greatest stake in the result, and this propels them to be more effective members of the rehabilitation team. When patients leave the operating room, they know exactly what they need to do to get a good result. What is more important, they know what they must *not* do. They know they can *move* the fingers, but that they cannot *use* the fingers or they will lose the good result.

- The therapist can also participate with the surgeon in intraoperative patient evaluation and education if invited into the operating room, as we do at our hospital (see Chapter 15).

- For a clip on a surgeon and therapist explaining the Saint John postoperative flexor tendon repair protocol to a patient during surgery, see Clip 15-3 in Chapter 15.

- Patients get to see that the repaired tendon works as they watch themselves moving the fingers through a full range of motion before the skin is closed. They know that their finger will function well once they get past the postoperative discomfort and stiffness if they put the effort into therapy.

- You and the hand therapist can get to know patients during the surgery and decide whether you can trust them with early protected movement.

WALANT ALLOWS YOU TO DETERMINE WHETHER SUPERFICIALIS REPAIR IS APPROPRIATE

- In a wide awake procedure you are able to have the patient move the hand through a full range of active movement.

- Based on this, you can repair the superficialis and see how this affects the full range of active movement during the surgery. If superficialis repair downgrades the movement, you can resect one of the slips or take down the whole superficialis repair to get the best possible active movement before you end the operation.

- For the full-length video of the repair of the 6-year-old patient shown in Clip 32-6, see Chapter 9, Clip 9-1. Also see Chapter 9, Clip 9-2, of a flexor tendon repair in a 10-year-old patient.

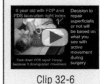

Clip 32-6
Determining
whether to repair the
superficialis.

OTHER ADVANTAGES OF WALANT VERSUS SEDATION AND TOURNIQUET

- A major advantage of eliminating sedation and the tourniquet for flexor tendon repair is that you do not need to perform the procedure in the main operating room. Some of us (authors) do all tendon repairs in minor procedure rooms in the clinic outside the main operating room Monday to Friday, 8 AM to 4 PM (see Chapter 16). Others of us still prefer to perform flexor tendon repair in the main operating room.

- We no longer need to perform such procedures at night. We know that we do better tendon repairs at 2 PM when we are fresh and awake than at 2 AM, when we are tired and sleepy.

- We no longer have to admit patients because of their medical comorbidities, which are only a problem when we sedate them.

- We perform the surgery with field sterility or add gowns and drapes for augmented field sterility (see Chapter 10).

- Working outside the main operating room also allows our hand therapists to be there to teach patients during the surgery and see the repair (see Chapter 15).

- You can suture the tendon inside the flexor sheath through sheathotomies to get a 1 cm bite without having to cut long segments of sheath when patients are wide awake (see the Tips and Tricks section). You can do this because you then test active flexion to prove that you have not caught your needle and suture inside the sheath.

- All of the general advantages listed in Chapter 2 apply to both the surgeon and the patient.

WHERE TO INJECT THE LOCAL ANESTHETIC FOR FLEXOR TENDON REPAIR OF THE FINGER

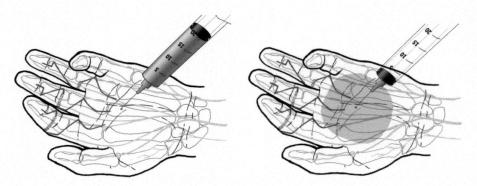

Inject 10 ml of 1% lidocaine with 1:100,000 epinephrine buffered with sodium bicarbonate (1 ml of 8.4% bicarbonate for each 10 ml of 1% lidocaine with 1:100,000 epinephrine) in the most proximal injection point. The first few milliliters go under the skin, and the rest is injected under the superficial palmar fascia without moving the needle. Wait 30 minutes for the local anesthesia to numb the common digital nerves, and then inject the distal palm (3 ml at each finger base) and fingers for the epinephrine effect. (From Lalonde DH, Kozin S. Tendon disorders of the hand. Plast Reconstr Surg 128:1e, 2011.)

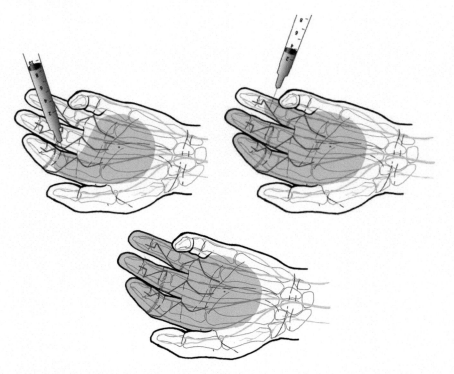

Inject 2 ml in the fat just below the skin between the two digital nerves in each of the proximal and middle phalanges. Inject one milliliter of the same solution in the subcutaneous fat in the middle of the distal phalanx just past the crease if you feel you will need to dissect in the distal phalanx. (From Lalonde DH, Kozin S. Tendon disorders of the hand. Plast Reconstr Surg 128:1e, 2011.)

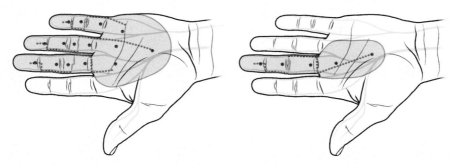

Alternative rectangular flap incisions are shown, which cover the tendon more effectively if the wounds dehisce. Some surgeons prefer to use only parts of the possible incisions illustrated.

- See Chapter 1, Atlas, for more illustrations of the anatomy of diffusion of tumescent local anesthetic in the forearm, wrist, and hand.

SPECIFICS OF MINIMALLY PAINFUL INJECTION OF LOCAL ANESTHETIC IN FLEXOR TENDON REPAIR OF THE FINGER

- Inject local anesthetic into the hand in the waiting area 30 or more minutes before surgery, as outlined in Chapters 4, 5, and 14. This allows the epinephrine to take effect and provides an adequately dry working field.[3]

- We inject patients while they are lying down to decrease the risk of their fainting (see Chapter 6).

- Use nonrefrigerated 1% lidocaine with 1:100,000 epinephrine buffered with 10 ml:1 ml of 8.4% sodium bicarbonate for all injections.

- During the injection, encourage the patient to look away. Create sensory "noise" to decrease pain by using pressure, touch, or pinch just proximal to the injection site. In the first injection, insert the needle perpendicular to the skin into the subcutaneous fat. Have your thumb ready on the plunger. Immobilize the syringe with fingers propped on the skin to avoid painful needle movement until the needle penetration site is numb.

- Start by injecting with a 27-gauge needle into the most proximal location that you are likely to find the proximal tendon stumps. For finger tendon lacerations, this usually means the proximal palm at the level at which the median nerve begins branching. If the injury disrupted the vincula and the proximal tendon flips proximally with great force out of the sheath and into the palm, you can retrieve it easily from the numbed palm.

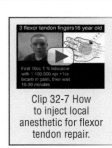

Clip 32-7 How to inject local anesthetic for flexor tendon repair.

- Inject the first 0.5 ml until it is visible below the skin, then pause. The first bleb must be visible or palpable under the skin to properly numb the needle insertion site. Wait 15 to 45 seconds until the patient tells you that the sting is gone. Then inject the rest of the 10 ml infiltration very slowly (over 2 to 3 minutes) without moving the needle.

- There is no need to move the needle distally as you inject. If you keep your needle in one place and continue to inject slowly, you will see and palpate the local anesthetic going everywhere in the palm. You want the area you will dissect to become a little firm with visible and palpable local anesthetic. You will not cause a palmar compartment syndrome. As soon as you incise the skin, the pressure will come down as the local anesthetic leaks out.

- If you inject 10 to 20 ml into the palm, where is it going to go? Everywhere! It is like an extravascular Bier block, but only where you need it.

- The goal of the injection is to bathe visible and palpable local anesthetic 2 cm beyond wherever you think you have even a small chance of dissecting.

- Wait 30 or more minutes if possible to let the palm's common digital nerves become completely numb. Then inject the distal palm with 3 ml at the base of each finger. After this, inject each proximal and middle phalanx with only 2 ml of buffered lidocaine and epinephrine in the subcutaneous fat between both digital nerves. The distal phalanges only get 1 ml between the digital nerves if dissection will be needed there. These finger injections are for the epinephrine effect.

IF YOU ARE WORKING WITH AN ANESTHESIOLOGIST

- Ask him or her to use only propofol. Inject the lidocaine with epinephrine as soon as the propofol permits pain-free injection of local anesthesia. The anesthesiologist can then wake the patient right away while you are scrubbing, prepping, and draping so you can get the benefit of intraoperative patient teaching (Chapter 8) and fully cooperative pain-free movement. This will give the epinephrine a little time to become more effective. Suggest that the anesthesia provider avoid administering opiates and amnestics to prevent nausea and permit the patient to remember your intraoperative advice. Patients will also remember the range of motion they can achieve.

TIPS AND TRICKS FOR PERFORMING FLEXOR TENDON REPAIR OF THE FINGER WITH THE WIDE AWAKE APPROACH

- When you are pulling the proximal tendon stump distally, an awake patient may find it hard to relax and may pull the tendon away from you. Ask the patient to extend the fingers while you flex the wrist and MP joints. Active extension of the fingers causes a spinal reflex relaxation of the finger flexors to help you deliver the tendon without extra incisions.

- Patients need to look at their fingers to know whether they are moving because they cannot feel them. However, if patients look, they can move just as they wish. Although most patients do not mind looking at the wound, you can cover it with a towel as they flex their fingers.

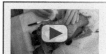

Clip 32-8 Dr. Jeffrey Yao has the patient see the fingers flex and extend.

- Consider accessing the tendon through a proximal sheathotomy where you can see it through the sheath. Leave the tendon in the sheath and push it with two Adson forceps. Thus you avoid having the forceps crush the severed tendon ends you are trying to heal. Alternatively (as preferred by Jin Bo Tang), the incision made to expose the tendon cut site can be quite short, and a separate small incision is made at the distal palm to find the retracted tendon, which is delivered through the intact sheath distally.

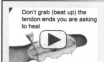

Clip 32-9 Retrieving the tendon from the proximal flexor sheath.

- You are more likely to keep the FDP between the two slips of the flexor digitorum superficialis (FDS) if you push it from proximal to distal than if you pass a red rubber catheter proximally and blindly down the sheath from the laceration site. However, even when you push the tendon from a proximal sheathotomy, it may not end up between the superficialis slips. Be sure you have restored that anatomy before you suture the tendon.

- Clip 32-10 shows an entire FDP repair with a four-strand locking Kessler repair and an epitenon suture (which is illustrated in Clip 32-11).

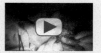

Clip 32-10 Delivering a misdirected FDP proximal stump between both slips of FDS.

- You can suture the tendon inside the flexor sheath through sheathotomies to get a 1 cm bite without having to cut long segments of sheath when the patient is wide awake (see the tips on pp. 194 and 195). You can do this because you can then test active flexion to prove that you have not caught your needle and suture inside the sheath. Use 3-0 or 4-0 sutures for core suture repair and 6-0 for peripheral suturing.

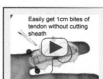

Clip 32-11 Suturing tendon inside flexor tendon sheath.

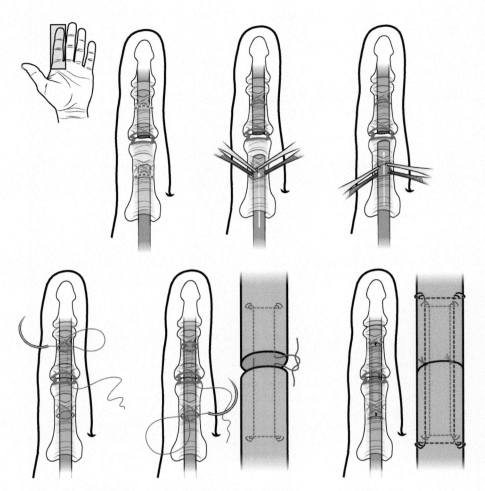

Retrieve the proximal tendon by performing a sheathotomy where you can see it through the sheath. Do not grab and crush the tendon ends you are going to ask to heal. Push the tendon forward in small increments by grabbing the tendon on the sides with two Adson forceps. Repair the tendon through the sheathotomies. Verify that you have not caught your needle with active flexion and extension. Repair the sheathotomies with an absorbable suture. These images show a four-strand locking Kessler with an epitenon repair. You can also use a six-strand M-shaped Jin Bo Tang repair using looped sutures or other repair with a simple running epitenon repair, not repairing the incised sheath.[4]

- Some of the authors of this chapter prefer less invasive exposure of the flexor sheath in the finger. They would rather make a separate incision in the palm and possibly advance the tendon from there using a pediatric feeding tube.[5]

- After the repair, ask the patient to make a full fist and extend the fingers completely. This is an important test to verify that the repair

is strong and can tolerate early active motion. The three parts of the digital extension-flexion test are:
1. Full active extension to verify no gapping between the tendon ends
2. Smooth active flexion to verify smooth gliding of the repair site
3. Total active flexion to verify that none of the pulleys prevents tendon gliding

- If the extension-flexion test creates a visible gap between the two tendon ends during finger extension, the suture is usually not tight enough and needs repair with additional tighter sutures with proper tension to avoid rupture. You can remove, tighten, or leave the previously loose suture, as appropriate. Slightly tensioning the repair is very important to prevent gapping.

- Do not be afraid to test full fist flexion and full extension. Your sutures need to be strong enough to take it. If they are not, you need to reinforce them. Repeated evaluation of total active movement is important to verify that the repair is strong and pulley release is sufficient.

- If active flexion indicates that the annular pulleys prevent the tendon from ample gliding, you can incrementally vent the pulleys until the patient achieves a full range of active motion before you close the skin. You can vent one half to two thirds of the distal part of the A2 pulley, and you can cut the entire A4 pulley and not get clinically significant bowstringing if adjacent pulleys are intact.

- Clip 32-12 shows total A4 pulley venting with no bowstringing with intraoperative total movement examination, and no bowstringing 6 months postoperatively. (See also Clip 15-1 in Chapter 15 of a tendon repair on a 10-year-old patient with venting of A3 and A4 pulleys and no bowstringing.)

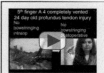

Clip 32-12 Total A4 pulley venting with no bowstringing.

- We do not worry about minor bleeding when we cut the skin, because most little bleeders will stop spontaneously by the time we sew the flaps to the dorsal skin for exposure. We no longer use cautery for most cases but occasionally use a hemostat on bigger veins for a few minutes.

- We always test flexor pollicis longus repairs as well as finger repairs to make certain there is no gapping and that the repair fits through the pulleys.

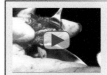

Clip 32-13 Testing flexor pollicis longus repair during surgery.

- To avoid numbness in the fingertip after dissection in zone 1 flexor tendon injuries, remember that 90% of the digital nerve goes to the fingertip. You want to make incisions midline in the volar pulp of the fingertip only as far as the center of the whorl of the fingerprint. Spread with scissors proximal to distal to the center of the whorl to avoid damaging the "leaves of the tree" of the digital nerves.

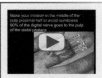

Clip 32-14 Where and how to dissect in pulp of distal phalanx to avoid numbness.

THE POSTOPERATIVE REGIMEN

- For more important details of the postoperative regimen for flexor tendon repair, see the following three videos: (1) Clip 32-4, in which the surgeon gets the confidence to allow the hand therapist to teach the patient up to half a fist of true active movement postoperatively, (2) Clip 32-5, in which intraoperative patient education decreases rupture and tenolysis rates, and (3) Clip 15-3 in Chapter 15 on the Saint John postoperative movement protocol for lacerated finger flexor tendons.

- The hand is elevated and not moved for the first 2 to 5 days to allow internal bleeding to stop. Moving the hand on the day of surgery causes internal bleeding, which results in edema and inflammation to remove the clot. The clot then turns to scar. There is no collagen formation in the first 3 days, so there is no need to move the fingers during that time. Elevation and immobilization for a few days will also allow any swelling to decrease and therefore decrease the work and friction of flexion, which decreases the risk of rupture.

- We want our patients off all pain medication when they start early protected movement so they know what hurts. We tell them to stop moving when they feel pain and listen to their body.

- We move the fingers passively before we move them actively to decrease joint friction and work of movement.

- All of the authors of this chapter use a similar form of postoperative early protected true active movement. They know that the patient was able to make a full fist and fully extend the fingers on the operating table without gapping. Good common sense tells us that up to half a fist of true active movement 3 days later will not cause a gap or rupture.

- Half a fist of early active movement makes the profundus glide 1 cm.

- Do *not* ask a patient to make a *full* fist with "place-and-hold" or true active movement therapy after surgery, because this can cause the repair to catch on the proximal edge of a hard pulley at 90 degrees, which can cause a gap in the repair. Instead, allow up to *half* a fist (45 degrees of flexion of the MP, PIP, and DIP joints) with early protected movement. You just want to keep the repair moving a little so it does not get stuck.

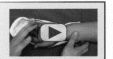

Clip 32-15 Passive and active finger movement up to half a fist after surgery.

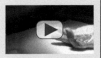

Clip 32-16 Profundus glides 1 cm of tendon when patient makes half a fist.

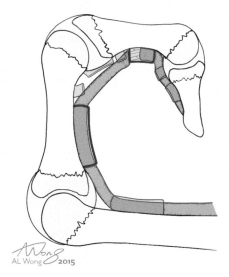

AL Wong 2015

Intraoperative full active fist testing reveals a gap caused by the tendon repair caught on the proximal edge of the hard entry point of the A4 pulley. This is a reason to avoid full-fist place-and-hold in postoperative therapy, which would have gone on to rupture. Other reasons are the highest work of flexion and highest friction with a full fist. Up to half a fist in postoperative active flexion is safer. When you see this gap with full fist testing at surgery, simply add sutures to the repair and vent the A4 pulley until you get full fist flexion with no gap.

- Clip 32-17 shows a tendon repair that caught on the proximal edge of the A4 pulley, causing a gap with full fist flexion. The gap was revealed and repaired during surgery. The A4 pulley was divided and the gap repaired before skin closure to avoid rupture.

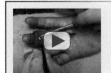

Clip 32-17 Tendon repair caught on proximal edge of A4 pulley.

References

1. Higgins A, Lalonde DH, Bell M, McKee D, Lalonde JF. Avoiding flexor tendon repair rupture with intraoperative total active movement examination. Plast Reconstr Surg 126:941, 2010.
2. Lalonde DH, Kozin S. Tendon disorders of the hand. Plast Reconstr Surg 128:1e, 2011.
3. McKee DE, Lalonde DH, Thoma A, Glennie DL, Hayward JE. Optimal time delay between epinephrine injection and incision to minimize bleeding. Plast Reconstr Surg 131:811, 2013.
4. Tang JB. Wide-awake primary flexor tendon repair, tenolysis, and tendon transfer. Clin Orthop Surg 7:275, 2015.
5. Wong J, McGrouther DA. Minimizing trauma over 'no man's land' with flexor tendon retrieval. J Hand Surg Eur 39:1004, 2014.

Clip 32-18 Fiona Peck Manchester short splint and Gwen van Strien scratch movement for true active movement after flexor tendon repair.

CHAPTER 33

FLEXOR TENDON REPAIR OF THE HAND

Donald H. Lalonde

ADVANTAGES OF WALANT VERSUS SEDATION AND TOURNIQUET IN FLEXOR TENDON REPAIR OF THE HAND

- The surgeon is less likely to have to perform secondary surgery for rupture repair if he or she tests the repair by having the patient take the fingers through a full range of motion before skin closure. If the surgeon sees gapping with the stress of full active movement, this can be repaired, with retesting of the repair to confirm that it is solid, and then the skin can be closed.[1] This is like testing and ensuring good patency and blood flow through a microvascular anastomosis before skin closure.

- See Chapter 32 for relevant videos, illustrations, and discussion of finger flexor tendon repairs.

- A major advantage of eliminating sedation for flexor tendon repair is that you do not need to perform the procedure in the main operating room. We do all of our tendon repairs in minor procedure rooms in the clinic outside the main operating room Monday to Friday, 8 AM to 4 PM. We know that we do better surgery at 2 PM than at 2 AM. In addition, our hand therapists can teach patients during the surgery and see the repair (see Chapter 15).

- You get to educate unsedated patients for the 90 or so minutes of the procedure without interruption. You can tell them that they can move their fingers but not use them, as the therapist will instruct. The patients will remember what you say and be even more motivated to follow hand therapy advice.

- Patients get to see that the repaired tendon works as they watch themselves moving their fingers through a full range of motion before skin closure. They know that their fingers will function well once they get past the postoperative discomfort and stiffness if they put the necessary effort into therapy.

- All of the general advantages listed in Chapters 2 and 32 apply to both the surgeon and the patient.

WHERE TO INJECT THE LOCAL ANESTHETIC FOR FLEXOR TENDON REPAIR OF THE HAND

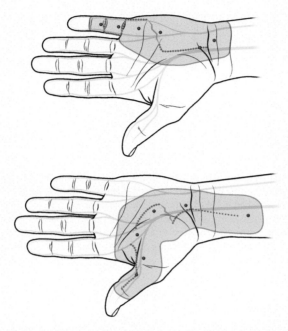

The orange lines represent the laceration and the dotted red lines are the possible incisions. This operation may benefit from a median/ulnar nerve block of 10 ml of 1% lidocaine with 1:100,000 epinephrine and 1 ml of 8.4% sodium bicarbonate under the skin and under the distal forearm fascia in the proximal red injection point. Up to 20 ml of the same solution would go in the palm, starting with 10 ml over the carpal tunnel, then 10 ml in the distal palm, and 2 ml in the proximal phalanx just under the skin. If the middle phalanx also needs exposure, you can inject another 2 ml there. The flexor pollicis longus (FPL) laceration shown in the carpal tunnel in the lower illustration above may benefit from a median nerve block of 10 ml of 1% lidocaine with 1:100,000 epinephrine and 1 ml of 8.4% sodium bicarbonate under the skin and under the distal forearm fascia in the proximal red injection point. Up to 20 ml of the same solution would go in the palm, starting with 10 ml over the carpal tunnel, then 10 ml over the thenar eminence and 2 ml in the thumb proximal phalanx injection point just under the skin. (Clip 43-9 in Chapter 43 shows this case.)

- See Chapter 1, Atlas, for more illustrations of the anatomy of diffusion of tumescent local anesthetic in the forearm, wrist, and hand.

SPECIFICS OF MINIMALLY PAINFUL INJECTION OF LOCAL ANESTHETIC IN FLEXOR TENDON REPAIR OF THE HAND

- Inject local anesthetic into the patient's hand in the waiting area 30 minutes before surgery. This allows the epinephrine to take effect and provides an adequately dry working field.[2]

- We inject patients while they are lying down on a stretcher to decrease the risk of their fainting (see Chapter 6).

- Use nonrefrigerated 1% lidocaine with 1:100,000 epinephrine buffered with 10:1 8.4% sodium bicarbonate for all injections. Keep the total dose of infiltration less than 7 mg/kg. If less than 50 ml will be required for tumescent local anesthesia (see Chapter 4), use premixed 1% lidocaine with 1:100,000 epinephrine. If 50 to 100 ml is required, dilute 50 ml of lidocaine and epinephrine with 50 ml of saline solution to produce a concentration of 0.5% lidocaine with 1:200,000 epinephrine.

- Flexor tendon lacerations of the hand frequently benefit from wrist median/ulnar nerve blocks. Start by injecting with a fine 27-gauge needle (not a 25-gauge) into the most proximal red injection point. Slowly inject 2 ml under the skin and then 8 ml under the forearm fascia to block the nerves.

- During the injection, encourage the patient to look away. Create sensory "noise" to decrease pain by using pressure, touch, or pinch near the injection site. In the first injection, insert the needle perpendicular to the skin into the subcutaneous fat. Immobilize the syringe with fingers propped on the skin to avoid the pain of needle wobble until the needle penetration site is numb. Inject the first 0.5 ml bleb slowly (5 seconds) and then pause. Wait 15 to 45 seconds until the patient tells you that all the sting is gone. Then inject the rest of the infiltrate very slowly (2 to 3 minutes) without moving the needle.

- There is no need to move the needle distally as you inject, only from superficial to below the wrist/forearm fascia. You will not cause a palmar compartment syndrome. As soon as you incise the skin, the pressure will come down as the local anesthetic leaks out.

- When performing major nerve blocks such as of the median or ulnar nerves, do not elicit paresthesias. Let the tumescent local anesthetic find and bathe the nerve so you do not damage it with the sharp needle tip.

- After the initial wrist median/ulnar nerve block, inject an additional 10 ml over the carpal tunnel superficial palmar fascia.

- Inject 10 ml under the skin of the thenar eminence. It will bathe the whole thenar pad, as shown in the thumb midmetacarpal volar illustration in Chapter 1.

- The goal of the injection is to bathe visible and palpable local anesthetic 2 cm beyond wherever you think you have even a small chance of dissecting in the wrist and hand.

- If you inject 20 ml into the palm, where will it go? Everywhere! Perfect! This is like an extravascular Bier block, but only where you need it.

- The metacarpal phalangeal crease of the thumb has sheath/cutaneous ligaments that are a natural barrier to the diffusion of local anesthetic into the proximal phalanx. Inject into the thenar eminence first to anesthetize the digital nerves of the proximal phalanx so the patient does not feel pain when you insert the needle into the thumb. Inject a further 2 ml into the subcutaneous fat in the proximal phalanx for the epinephrine effect in case the distal end of FPL or FDP is there.

IF YOU ARE WORKING WITH AN ANESTHESIOLOGIST

- Ask him or her to use only propofol. Inject the lidocaine with epinephrine as soon as the propofol permits pain-free injection of local anesthetic. This will give the epinephrine a little time to become more effective. The anesthesiologist can then wake the patient right away while you are scrubbing, prepping, and draping so you can get the benefit of intraoperative patient teaching (Chapter 8) and fully cooperative pain-free movement. Suggest that the anesthesia provider avoid administering opiates and amnestics to prevent nausea and permit the patient to remember your intraoperative advice. Patients will also remember the range of motion they can achieve.

TIPS AND TRICKS FOR DOING FLEXOR TENDON REPAIR OF THE HAND WITH THE WIDE AWAKE APPROACH

- Do not worry about minor bleeding from cut skin edges, because most little bleeders will stop spontaneously by the time you finish tacking the skin flaps back for exposure. We no longer use cautery for flexor tendon repairs but occasionally use a hemostat on bigger vessels for a few minutes.

- When you are delivering the proximal tendon into the wound, it is helpful to ask the patient to try to relax the flexors. It is even more helpful to ask the patient to extend the fingers while you flex the wrist and MP joints. Active extension of the fingers causes a spinal reflex relaxation of the finger flexors to help you deliver them into the wound without extra incisions.

- Patients need to look at their fingers to get them to move. They cannot feel their numbed finger move, because it has lost its proprioceptive sense. However, if patients look, they can move the finger just as they wish. Although many patients do not mind looking at the wound, you can cover the wound with a towel as they flex the fingers or thumb while looking at them.

- Do not be afraid to test full flexion and full extension. Your sutures need to be strong enough to take flexion and extension. If they are not, you need to reinforce them.

- See Clip 43-9 in Chapter 43 of an original repair and subsequent ruptured FPL repair under the motor branch in the carpal tunnel.

- See the many additional tips and tricks of flexor tendon repair in Chapter 32.

References

1. Higgins A, Lalonde DH, Bell M, McKee D, Lalonde JF. Avoiding flexor tendon repair rupture with intraoperative total active movement examination. Plast Reconstr Surg 126:941, 2010.
2. McKee DE, Lalonde DH, Thoma A, Glennie DL, Hayward JE. Optimal time delay between epinephrine injection and incision to minimize bleeding. Plast Reconstr Surg 131:811, 2013.

CHAPTER 34
FLEXOR TENDON REPAIR OF THE FOREARM

Donald H. Lalonde

ADVANTAGES OF WALANT VERSUS SEDATION AND TOURNIQUET IN FLEXOR TENDON REPAIR OF THE FOREARM

- Many of these injuries happen at night and on weekends—not an ideal time to perform a repair. WALANT permits the elective scheduling of these operations in minor procedure rooms outside the main operating room Monday through Friday, 8 AM to 4 PM, after the wound is washed and the skin is closed in the emergency department. This permits patients to be sober so they can understand their injury and learn how to look after it with intraoperative teaching they can remember.

- We all do better surgery at 11 AM than at 11 PM.

- It is often difficult to tell which proximal tendon stumps belong to which distal tendons in a "spaghetti wrist" injury. This can be even more difficult with ragged cuts such as might happen with a table saw accident. If you ask the patient to flex the long finger, the proximal long finger profundus and superficialis tendon stumps move the most. This helps you in tendon identification and correct matching of proximal to distal structures (see Clip 34-1).

- You can ask the patient to move each finger, and you will see which proximal tendons belong to which distal tendons, because comfortable tourniquet-free patients can control the movement of the proximal stumps.

Clip 34-1 "Spaghetti wrist." Active movement in proximal forearm identifies which proximal tendons belong to which distal tendon ends.

- You can educate your patients during the case about how important it is that they keep their hand elevated and "on strike," doing absolutely nothing with it for the next week while the tendons heal. At the end of the procedure, they sit up and elevate their hand with total understanding of what to do. If they had been asleep, they might not understand as well what they should do after surgery. They may keep their hand dependent and are more likely to try to use their fingers and hand.

- All of the general advantages listed in Chapters 2 and 32 apply to both the surgeon and the patient.

WHERE TO INJECT THE LOCAL ANESTHETIC FOR FLEXOR TENDON REPAIR OF THE FOREARM

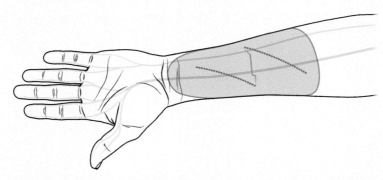

The orange line in the illustration is the laceration and the dotted red lines are the possible incisions. Inject up to 100 ml of 0.5% lidocaine with 1:200,000 (buffered with 10 ml of 1% lidocaine with 1:100,000 epinephrine:1 ml of 8.4% sodium bicarbonate). Add 10 ml 0.5% bupivacaine with 1:200,000 epinephrine to the injectate if you think the procedure will take more than 2½ hours.

- See Chapter 1, Atlas, for more illustrations of the anatomy of diffusion of tumescent local anesthetic in the forearm, wrist, and hand.

SPECIFICS OF MINIMAL PAIN INJECTION OF LOCAL ANESTHETIC IN FLEXOR TENDON REPAIR OF THE FOREARM

- Inject the anesthetic solution a minimum of 30 minutes before surgery to allow the epinephrine to take optimal effect and provide an adequately dry working field,[1] as outlined in Chapters 4 and 14.
- We inject supine patients lying down on stretchers in a waiting area to decrease the risk of their fainting (see Chapter 6).
- Use nonrefrigerated 1% lidocaine with 1:100,000 epinephrine buffered with 10:1 8.4% bicarbonate for all injections. Keep the total dose of infiltration less than 7 mg/kg. If less than 50 ml will be required, use premixed 1% lidocaine with 1:100,000 epinephrine. If 50 to 100 ml is required, dilute with saline solution to a concentration of 0.5% lidocaine with 1:200,000 epinephrine. If 100 to 200 ml of solution is required to produce tumescent local anesthesia (see Chapter 4), dilute with saline solution to a concentration of 0.25% lidocaine with 1:400,000 epinephrine.
- To minimize the pain of injection, start to inject with a fine 27-gauge needle (not a 25-gauge) 2 cm proximal to the most proximal place you are likely to dissect.
- Ask the patient to look away. Press with a fingertip just proximal to the injection site before you put in the needle to add the sensory

"noise" of pressure to decrease the pain. The skin of the volar forearm is loose, so you can pinch it gently and push the skin into the needle as another technique to reduce needle insertion pain.

- Insert the first needle perpendicularly into the subcutaneous fat. Stabilize the syringe with two hands to avoid the pain of needle wobble until the skin needle site is numb. Inject the first visible 0.5 ml bleb, then pause. Wait 15 to 45 seconds until the patient tells you that all the needle pain is gone. Inject the rest of the first 10 ml slowly (over 2 minutes) without moving the needle.

- Reinsert the needle farther distally into skin that is within 1 cm of clearly vasoconstricted white skin that has functioning lidocaine and epinephrine so that needle reinsertion is pain free.

- Continue injecting from proximal to distal, blowing the local anesthetic slowly ahead of the needle so there is always at least 1 cm of visible or palpable local anesthesia ahead of the sharp needle tip point that the patient would feel if you advanced it into "live" nerves. "Blow slow before you go." (See Chapter 5 for further tips on how to inject the local anesthesia with minimal pain.)

- The goal of the injection is to bathe local anesthetic 2 cm beyond wherever you think you even have a small chance of dissecting in the forearm.

- Most of the injection is in the subcutaneous plane. After the skin flaps are elevated and you identify the plane between superficialis and profundus, an additional 20 ml of local in this plane will numb the median nerve indirectly. Alternatively, you can elevate the superficialis muscle, identify the median and/or ulnar nerves, and slowly inject 5 ml of local anesthetic into the loose areolar tissue around the nerve or nerves. Do not inject directly into the nerves, as you will lacerate fascicles and damage axons.

- The more volume that you inject, the greater are the odds that the patient will feel no pain after you begin dissection. Try to avoid "top-ups" of local anesthetic that give patients unnecessary bad memories.

- If you have access to blunt-tipped injection cannulas such as those used to inject dermal fillers, you can inject the local anesthetic painlessly more quickly than with a sharp needle tip[2] (see Chapter 5).

IF YOU ARE WORKING WITH AN ANESTHESIOLOGIST

- Ask him or her to use only propofol. Inject the lidocaine with epinephrine as soon as the propofol permits pain-free injection of local anesthesia. This will give the epinephrine a little time to become more effective. The anesthesiologist can then wake the patient right away while you are scrubbing, prepping, and draping so you can get the benefit of intraoperative patient teaching (Chapter 8) and fully cooperative pain-free movement. Suggest that the anesthesia provider avoid administering opiates and amnestics to prevent nausea and permit patients to remember your intraoperative advice. Patients will also remember the range of motion they can achieve.

TIPS AND TRICKS FOR PERFORMING FLEXOR TENDON REPAIR OF THE FOREARM WITH THE WIDE AWAKE APPROACH

- See the many additional tips and tricks for flexor tendon repair in Chapter 32.

- We do not worry about minor bleeding from cut skin edges, because most little bleeders will stop spontaneously by the time we sew the skin flaps back for exposure. We no longer use cautery but occasionally use a hemostat on larger veins for a few minutes, or we tie them off.

- We use augmented field sterility in our minor procedure rooms for longer cases such as these by importing full drapes and gowns from the main operating room (see Chapter 10).

- We wait for at least 30 minutes between local anesthetic injection in the patient waiting area and bringing the patient into the minor procedure room to allow the epinephrine to reach maximal vasoconstriction. We perform a couple of carpal tunnels or see patients for hand consultations from the emergency department while waiting so our time is used productively.

- We ask patients to go to the restroom to relieve themselves after we inject the local anesthetic and just before we start the surgery to avoid unnecessary surgical interruptions for these longer cases. The patient has no intravenous infusion that would increase the urge to void. If we give preoperative antibiotics, they are administered by mouth.

- When you are trying retrieve or to sew the tendons together, the patient may pull the proximal tendons away from you. If you ask him or her to extend the fingers, the flexor muscles reflexly relax and the patient will stop pulling as much. In addition, you can keep the wrist and fingers passively flexed, which will also help to decrease the tension on the repair.

References

1. McKee DE, Lalonde DH, Thoma A, Glennie DL, Hayward JE. Optimal time delay between epinephrine injection and incision to minimize bleeding. Plast Reconstr Surg 131:811, 2013.
2. Lalonde D, Wong A, Local anesthetics: What's new in minimal pain injection and best evidence in pain control. Plast Reconstr Surg 134(4 Suppl 2):40S, 2014.

CHAPTER 35

EXTENSOR TENDON REPAIR OF THE FINGER

Donald H. Lalonde

ADVANTAGES OF WALANT VERSUS SEDATION AND TOURNIQUET IN EXTENSOR TENDON REPAIR OF THE FINGER

- You can simulate the relative motion extension splint during WALANT surgery with a sterile tongue depressor.[1-3] This will help you decide whether you need to add a wrist component to the Merritt splint. Wyndell Merritt's relative motion extension splint has revolutionized management of lacerations at the proximal phalanx and dorsal hand levels (see Chapter 37) in the last few years. Patients can return to work with these very functional splints as early as a few days after surgery.

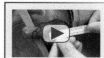
Clip 35-1 Relative motion extension splint decreases excursion in extensor tendon repair in the proximal finger.

- Clip 35-1 demonstrates that the relative motion extension splint decreases excursion in extensor tendon repair in the proximal finger. The relative motion extension splint keeps the MP joint of the affected finger more extended than the other MP joints. This takes the tension off the long extensors, even when fingers are actively flexing. (See also video clips in Chapter 37.)

- You can simulate the relative motion flexion splint during WALANT boutonniere surgery or in clinic consultations with a sterile tongue depressor. The Merritt relative motion flexion splint has revolutionized acute and chronic boutonniere management in the last few years. Patients can return to work with these very functional splints.

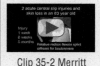
Clip 35-2 Merritt relative motion flexion splinting for boutonniere deformity.

- Clip 35-2 shows Merritt relative motion flexion splinting for boutonniere deformity. The relative motion flexion splint keeps the MP joint of the affected finger more flexed than the MP joints of the adjacent fingers. This increased tension on the long extensors pulls the lateral bands dorsal to the axis of the PIP joint while taking the tension off the intrinsic volar pull on the same lateral bands.

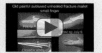
Clip 35-3 WALANT mallet fracture management.

- WALANT takes many of the inconveniences of general and motor block anesthesia out of the management of fracture mallet injuries.

- All of the general advantages listed in Chapter 2 apply to both the surgeon and the patient.

WHERE TO INJECT THE LOCAL ANESTHETIC FOR EXTENSOR TENDON REPAIR OF THE FINGER

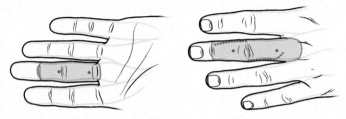

The orange line in the illustration is the laceration and the dotted red lines are the possible incisions. *Palmar injections:* Inject 2 ml of 1% lidocaine with 1:100,000 epinephrine (buffered with 10 ml lido/epi:1 ml of 8.4% sodium bicarbonate) in the most proximal red injection point in the subcutaneous palmar fat. Perform the most proximal dorsal injection next, and then inject 2 ml in the middle of the subcutaneous fat of the palmar middle phalanx. *Dorsal injections:* Inject 2 ml of 1% lidocaine with 1:100,000 epinephrine (buffered with 10 ml lido/epi:1 ml of 8.4% sodium bicarbonate) in the proximal red injection dot in the subcutaneous fat of the dorsal proximal phalanx. Inject the middle phalanx palmar side next and then finally inject 2 ml in the middle of the dorsal middle phalanx subcutaneous fat.

- See Chapter 1, Atlas, for more illustrations of the anatomy of diffusion of tumescent local anesthetic in the forearm, wrist, and hand.

SPECIFICS OF MINIMALLY PAINFUL INJECTION OF LOCAL ANESTHETIC IN EXTENSOR TENDON REPAIR OF THE FINGER

- Inject just under the skin. There is no need to inject into the sheath; this would only add unnecessary pain.

- Inject the anesthetic solution a minimum of 30 minutes before surgery to allow the epinephrine to take optimal effect and provide an adequately dry working field,[4] as outlined in Chapters 4 and 14.

- We inject supine patients lying down on stretchers in a waiting area before they come into the operating room to decrease the risk of their fainting (see Chapter 6).

- To minimize the pain of injection, use a 27-gauge needle (not a 25-gauge).

- Ask the patient to look away. Press with a fingertip just proximal to the injection site before you put in the needle to add the sensory "noise" of pressure to decrease the pain.

- Insert the first needle perpendicularly into the subcutaneous fat. Stabilize the syringe with two hands and have your thumb ready on the plunger to avoid the pain of needle wobble until the skin needle site is numb. Inject the first visible 0.5 ml bleb and then pause. Wait 15 to 45 seconds until the patient tells you that all the needle pain is gone. Inject the rest of the 2 ml slowly (over 1 minute) without moving the needle.

- In this operation, inject 2 ml in the palmar proximal phalanx first, then inject 2 ml in the dorsal proximal phalanx after that. This will give the local anesthetic time to numb the digital nerves proximally so the phalangeal injections will hurt less.

IF YOU ARE WORKING WITH AN ANESTHESIOLOGIST

- Ask him or her to use only propofol. Inject the lidocaine with epinephrine as soon as the propofol permits pain-free injection of local anesthetic. This will give the epinephrine a little time to become more effective. The anesthesiologist can then wake the patient right away while you are scrubbing, prepping, and draping so you can get the benefit of intraoperative patient teaching (Chapter 8) and fully cooperative pain-free movement. Suggest that the anesthesia provider avoid administering opiates and amnestics to prevent nausea and permit patients to remember your intraoperative advice. Patients will also remember the range of motion they can achieve.

TIPS AND TRICKS FOR PERFORMING EXTENSOR TENDON REPAIR OF THE FINGER WITH THE WIDE AWAKE APPROACH

- Percutaneous extensor tendon repair is useful because the thin finger extensor tendon does not hold a suture very well. Nylon sutures through both skin and tendon hold the suture better. This is especially true when the skin is frayed, such as from a table saw accident. The ends of the extensor tendon are close enough that the splinting will allow functional healing of the tendon with a gap.

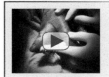

Clip 35-4
Percutaneous
extensor tendon
repair.

- You can see that your sutures are tight enough with WALANT, because the finger stays in full extension when you let it go and stop holding it up. Avoiding buried permanent sutures also avoids stitch abscesses later. For the past 10 years, I have mostly used monofilament absorbable suture on the extensor side of fingers if I use anything buried at all.

- Use the pencil test to simulate relative motion flexion and extension splints in the clinic when you evaluate patients with hand problems. It will help you solve many problems such as boutonniere deformity, extensor lag, flexor lag, interosseous muscle tear, and sagittal band rupture.

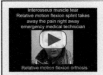

Clip 35-5 Pencil test
for relative motion
splinting.

- Patients may need to look at their fingers to get them to extend to test the repair, since they may not feel the numbed fingers. Although most patients do not mind looking at the wound, you can cover the wound with a towel as they watch their fingers move.

- In contrast to flexor tendon repairs, we do not make patients test extensor tendon repairs over the proximal phalanx with a full fist of flexion. The sutures will generally not hold well enough in the thin extensor tendons. Flexor tendon repairs are stronger and withstand full fist flexion testing easily. In addition, finger extensor repairs can tolerate a gap, as we all witness with most mallet injuries. Flexor tendon lacerations do not tolerate a gap.

- Many patients are interested in looking at the tendon to understand the nature of their problem. You can put a mask on the patient, show him the tendon and have him watch it move. Many patients love this type of thing. Some patients will tell others it is something they need to put on their bucket list!

- You can perform these operations with field sterility to increase efficiency (see Chapter 10).

References

1. Howell JW, Merritt WH, Robinson SJ. Immediate controlled active motion following zone 4-7 extensor tendon repair. J Hand Ther 18:182, 2005.
2. Merritt WH. Relative motion splint: active motion after extensor tendon injury and repair. J Hand Surg Am 39:1187, 2014.
3. Burns MC, Derby B, Neumeister MW. Wyndell Merritt immediate controlled active motion (ICAM) protocol following extensor tendon repairs in zone IV-VII: review of literature, orthosis design, and case study—a multimedia article. Hand (N Y) 8:17, 2013.
4. McKee DE, Lalonde DH, Thoma A, Glennie DL, Hayward JE. Optimal time delay between epinephrine injection and incision to minimize bleeding. Plast Reconstr Surg 131:811, 2013.

CHAPTER 36

EXTENSOR TENDON REPAIR OF THE HAND

Donald H. Lalonde, Geoff Cook

ADVANTAGES OF WALANT VERSUS SEDATION AND TOURNIQUET IN EXTENSOR TENDON REPAIR OF THE HAND

- You can see that that your repair is solid enough by watching the patient take the fingers through a full range of motion before you close the skin.

- You can simulate the relative motion extension splint during WALANT surgery with a sterile tongue depressor,[1-3] This will help you decide whether you need to add a wrist component to the Merritt splint. Wyndell Merritt's relative motion extension splint has revolutionized extensor tendon laceration of the proximal phalanx (see Clip 35-1 in Chapter 35) and dorsal hand management in the last few years. Patients can go back to work with these very functional splints as early as a few days after surgery, as shown in Clip 36-1.

- The relative motion extension splint keeps the MP joint of the affected finger more extended than the other MP joints. This takes the tension off the repaired long extensor, even when fingers are actively flexing.

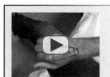

Clip 36-1 Hand extensor repair revolutionized by Merritt relative motion extension splinting.

- Patients get to see their finger movement restored during the surgery. They will remember this light at the end of the tunnel when they are working through the pain and stiffness of postoperative healing and therapy.

- All of the general advantages listed in Chapter 2 apply to both the surgeon and the patient.

WHERE TO INJECT THE LOCAL ANESTHETIC FOR EXTENSOR TENDON REPAIR OF THE HAND

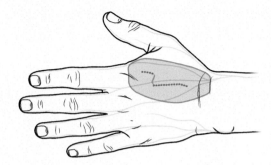

Inject 20 ml of 1% lidocaine with 1:100,000 epinephrine buffered with 2 ml of 8.4% sodium bicarbonate. The orange line in the illustration is the laceration and the dotted red lines are the possible incisions.

- See Chapter 1, Atlas, for more illustrations of the anatomy of diffusion of tumescent local anesthetic in the forearm, wrist, and hand.

SPECIFICS OF MINIMALLY PAINFUL INJECTION OF LOCAL ANESTHETIC IN EXTENSOR TENDON REPAIR OF THE HAND

- Inject the anesthetic solution a minimum of 30 minutes before surgery to allow the epinephrine to take optimal effect and provide an adequately dry working field,[4] as outlined in Chapters 4 and 14.

- We inject supine patients lying down on stretchers in a waiting area to decrease the risk of their fainting (see Chapter 6).

- To minimize the pain of injection, use a fine 27-gauge needle (not a 25-gauge).

- Ask the patient to look away. Press with a fingertip just proximal to the injection site before you put in the needle to add the sensory "noise" of pressure to decrease the pain. The skin of the dorsal hand is loose. You can therefore pinch it gently and push the skin into the needle as another technique to reduce needle insertion pain.

- Insert the first needle perpendicularly into the subcutaneous fat. Stabilize the syringe with two hands to avoid the pain of needle wobble until the skin needle site is numb. Inject the first visible 0.5 ml bleb and then pause. Wait 15 to 45 seconds until the patient tells you that all the needle pain is gone. Inject the rest of the first 10 ml slowly (over 2 minutes) without moving the needle.

- Reinsert the needle farther distally within 1 cm of clearly vasoconstricted white skin that has functioning lidocaine and epinephrine so the needle reinsertion is pain free.

- Continue injecting from proximal to distal, blowing the local anesthetic slowly ahead of the needle so there is always at least 1 cm of visible or palpable local anesthetic ahead of the sharp needle tip that the patient would feel if you advanced it into "live" nerves. "Blow slow before you go." (See Chapter 5 for further tips on how to inject the local anesthetic with minimal pain.)

- The goal of the injection is to get visible and palpable local anesthetic under the skin at least 2 cm outside any area you are likely to dissect.

- Keep the total dose of infiltration less than 7 mg/kg. If less than 50 ml will be required to produce tumescent local anesthesia (see Chapter 4), we use premixed 1% lidocaine with 1:100,000 epinephrine. If 50 to 100 ml is required, we dilute with saline solution to a concentration of 0.5% lidocaine with 1:200,000 epinephrine.

IF YOU ARE WORKING WITH AN ANESTHESIOLOGIST

- Ask him or her to use only propofol. Inject the lidocaine with epinephrine as soon as the propofol permits pain-free injection of local anesthetic. This will give the epinephrine a little time to become more effective. The anesthesiologist can then wake the patient right away while you are scrubbing, prepping, and draping so you can get the benefit of intraoperative patient teaching (Chapter 8) and fully cooperative pain-free movement. Suggest that the anesthesia provider avoid administering opiates and amnestics to prevent nausea and permit the patient to remember your intraoperative advice. Patients will also remember the range of motion they can achieve.

TIPS AND TRICKS FOR PERFORMING EXTENSOR TENDON REPAIR OF THE HAND WITH THE WIDE AWAKE APPROACH

- To get the extensors to relax, ask the patient to flex the finger. There is a reflex arc in the spinal cord that causes the extensors to relax.

- Test full fist flexion and full extension after every extensor tendon repair over the hand with the protection of a tongue depressor that simulates a relative motion extension splint, as shown in Clip 36-1. You can then have your therapists build a splint for the patient and begin early protected movement a few days after surgery in reliable patients.

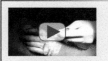
Clip 36-2 Extensors reflexively relax when patient is asked to actively flex the finger.

- Patients may need to look at their fingers to get them to extend to test the repair, since they may not feel the numbed fingers. Although most patients do not mind looking at the wound, you can cover the wound with a towel as they watch their fingers move.

- Many patients are interested in looking at the tendon to understand their problem. You can mask patients, show them the tendon, and have them watch it move. Many patients love this. Some patients will tell others it is something they need to put on their bucket list!

- You can perform this brief operation with field sterility to increase efficiency (Chapter 10). Alternatively, you may choose to bring drapes and gowns into the clinic for augmented field sterility.

References

1. Howell JW, Merritt WH, Robinson SJ. Immediate controlled active motion following zone 4-7 extensor tendon repair. J Hand Ther 18:182, 2005.
2. Merritt WH. Relative motion splint: active motion after extensor tendon injury and repair. J Hand Surg Am 39:1187, 2014.
3. Burns MC, Derby B, Neumeister MW. Wyndell Merritt immediate controlled active motion (ICAM) protocol following extensor tendon repairs in zone IV-VII: review of literature, orthosis design, and case study—a multimedia article. Hand (N Y) 8:17, 2013.
4. McKee DE, Lalonde DH, Thoma A, Glennie DL, Hayward JE. Optimal time delay between epinephrine injection and incision to minimize bleeding. Plast Reconstr Surg 131:811, 2013.

CHAPTER 37
EXTENSOR TENDON REPAIR OF THE FOREARM

Donald H. Lalonde

ADVANTAGES OF WALANT VERSUS SEDATION AND TOURNIQUET IN EXTENSOR TENDON REPAIR OF THE FOREARM

- You can test the strength of your forearm extensor tendon repairs by asking patients to make a fist and extend their fingers and wrist. If you see gapping, you can strengthen your repairs with more sutures to avoid rupture postoperatively.

- You can allow finger movement while patients recover from the tendon repair based on what you see with active movement during the surgery. You may put them into relative motion extension splinting, which you can simulate with a tongue depressor during the surgery (see Chapters 35 and 36).

- Patients can see that they can once again move their fingers without pain during the surgery. They know that they can get their movement back after they work through the pain and stiffness of the surgery.

- All of the general advantages listed in Chapter 2 apply to both the surgeon and the patient.

WHERE TO INJECT THE LOCAL ANESTHETIC FOR EXTENSOR TENDON REPAIR OF THE FOREARM

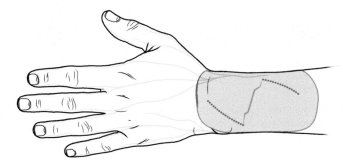

The orange line in the illustration is the laceration and the dotted red lines are the possible incisions. Inject up to 100 ml of 0.5% lidocaine with 1:200,000 epinephrine (buffered with 10 ml of 1% lidocaine with 1:100,000 epinephrine:1 ml of 8.4% sodium bicarbonate). Add 10 ml 0.5% bupivacaine with 1:200,000 epinephrine to the injectate if you think the procedure will take more than 2½ hours.

- See Chapter 1, Atlas, for more illustrations of the anatomy of diffusion of tumescent local anesthetic in the forearm, wrist, and hand.

SPECIFICS OF MINIMALLY PAINFUL INJECTION OF LOCAL ANESTHETIC IN EXTENSOR TENDON REPAIR OF THE FOREARM

- Inject the anesthetic solution a minimum of 30 minutes before surgery to allow the epinephrine to take optimal effect and provide an adequately dry working field,[1] as outlined in Chapters 4, 5, and 14.

- We inject supine patients lying down on stretchers in a waiting area to decrease the risk of their fainting (see Chapter 6).

- To minimize the pain of injection, use a small 27-gauge needle (not a 25-gauge).

- Ask the patient to look away. Press with a fingertip just proximal to the injection site before you put in the needle to add the sensory "noise" of pressure to decrease the pain. The skin of the dorsal forearm is loose. You can therefore pinch it gently and push the skin into the needle as another technique to reduce needle insertion pain.

- Insert the first needle perpendicularly into the subcutaneous fat. Stabilize the syringe with two hands and have your thumb ready on the plunger to avoid the pain of needle wobble until the skin needle site is numb. Inject the first visible 0.5 ml bleb and then pause. Wait 15 to 45 seconds until the patient tells you that all the needle pain is gone. Inject the rest of the first 10 ml slowly (over 2 to 3 minutes) without moving the needle.

- Continue injecting from proximal to distal, blowing the local anesthetic slowly ahead of the needle so there is always at least 1 cm of visible or palpable local anesthetic ahead of the sharp needle tip that the patient would feel if you advanced it into "live" nerves. "Blow slow before you go." (See Chapter 5 for further tips on how to inject the local anesthetic with minimal pain.)

- Reinsert the needle within 1 cm of clearly vasoconstricted white skin that has functioning lidocaine and epinephrine so the needle reinsertion is pain free.

- The goal of the injection is to bathe local anesthetic at least 2 cm outside of wherever you think you have even a small chance of dissecting in the forearm.

- If you have access to blunt-tipped injection cannulas,[2] you can inject the local anesthetic with minimal pain and quicker than with a sharp needle tip (see Chapter 5).

IF YOU ARE WORKING WITH AN ANESTHESIOLOGIST

- Ask him or her to use only propofol. Inject the lidocaine with epinephrine as soon as the propofol permits pain-free injection of local anesthetic. This will give the epinephrine a little time to become more effective. The anesthesiologist can then wake the patient right away while you are scrubbing, prepping, and draping so you can get the benefit of intraoperative patient teaching (Chapter 8) and fully cooperative pain-free movement. Suggest that the anesthesia provider avoid administering opiates and amnestics to prevent nausea and permit the patient to remember your intraoperative advice. Patients will also remember the range of motion they can achieve.

TIPS AND TRICKS FOR PERFORMING EXTENSOR TENDON REPAIR OF THE FOREARM WITH THE WIDE AWAKE APPROACH

- Clip 37-1 provides three different extensor tendon repairs of the forearm, including a case of primary tendon graft to EPL after rupture from a distal radius fracture.

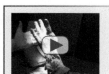

Clip 37-1 Three different extensor tendon repairs of the forearm.

- Do not worry about minor bleeding from cut skin edges, because most little bleeders will stop spontaneously by the time you sew the skin flaps back for exposure. We no longer use cautery for most cases but occasionally use a hemostat on bigger vessels for a few minutes, or tie them off.

- Patients may need to look at their fingers to get them to extend to test the repair, since they may not feel the numbed fingers. Although most patients do not mind looking at the wound, you can cover the wound with a towel as they watch their fingers move.

- It is worth placing a tongue depressor under the involved finger or fingers to perform the repair and to simulate a relative motion extension splint intraoperatively. This may allow you to let the patient have early protected movement of the fingers at 3 to 5 days after surgery[3,4] (see Chapters 35 and 36).

References

1. McKee DE, Lalonde DH, Thoma A, Glennie DL, Hayward JE. Optimal time delay between epinephrine injection and incision to minimize bleeding. Plast Reconstr Surg 131:811, 2013.
2. Lalonde D, Wong A. Local anesthetics: what's new in minimal pain injection and best evidence in pain control. Plast Reconstr Surg 134(4 Suppl 2):40S, 2014.
3. Howell JW, Merritt WH, Robinson SJ. Immediate controlled active motion following zone 4-7 extensor tendon repair. J Hand Ther 18:182, 2005.
4. Merritt WH. Relative motion splint: active motion after extensor tendon injury and repair. J Hand Surg Am 39:1187, 2014.

CHAPTER 38
TENOLYSIS

Jason Wong, Michael Sauerbier, Peter C. Amadio, Donald H. Lalonde

ADVANTAGES OF WALANT VERSUS SEDATION AND TOURNIQUET IN TENOLYSIS

- There is no rush when performing tenolysis, because there is no tourniquet.

- Your patients can help you, because they are comfortable and cooperative; they can rupture their own adhesions by actively flexing their muscles after you release some of the adhesions.

- Patients can show you where their tendon is stuck with active movement; sometimes the tendon stuck in a place that may surprise you.

- In Clip 38-1, Dr. Jason Wong performs tenolysis after a finger amputation. The patient, pain-free and cooperative, helps the surgeon rupture the last of the adhesions.

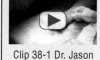
Clip 38-1 Dr. Jason Wong performs tenolysis after finger amputation.

- You will know that you finished the surgery when you see a full range of active finger movement while the patient is on the operating table. This is like testing and ensuring good patency and blood flow through a microvascular anastomosis before you close the skin.

- At the end of the surgery, you can show your patients exercises they can perform. They can do their first exercises on the table in a totally pain-free manner instead of after surgery, when they will be sore. They will remember the exercises and the range of motion they can achieve because they are sedation free.

- You and the patient will both know how much active movement the finger achieved at the end of the operation. This avoids unrealistic expectations for you and the patient.

- In Clip 38-2, Dr. Michael Sauerbier performs tenolysis with the wide awake approach. Thus the patient can remember the movement he was able to experience on the operating table.

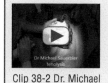
Clip 38-2 Dr. Michael Sauerbier performs tenolysis.

- Patients watch themselves moving the fingers through a full range of motion before the skin is closed. They know that their finger will function well once they get past the postoperative discomfort and stiffness if they put effort into their therapy.

- You are able to talk to unsedated patients for the 90 or so minutes that local anesthesia and the tenolysis take to accomplish. You can educate and warn them about what to do and not do after surgery. We know that the tendon is weaker and has less blood supply after tenolysis. Therefore, to avoid rupture we warn patients to avoid jerk-type movements and heavy lifting for 2 to 3 weeks until the tendon gets stronger.

- You can get to know your patients better during the surgery and find out what will motivate them. The patient in Clip 38-3 wanted to succeed in an Olympic sport. Seeing her finger move at surgery motivated her to maintain the movement after surgery.

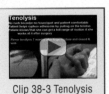

Clip 38-3 Tenolysis after finger fracture.

- The hand therapist can also participate in intraoperative patient evaluation and education if the surgeon allows the therapist into the operating room, as we do (see Chapter 15).

- All of the general advantages listed in Chapter 2 apply to both the surgeon and the patient.

WHERE TO INJECT THE LOCAL ANESTHETIC FOR TENOLYSIS

The orange line represents the patient's original scarring from 60 years before (see Clip 38-4). For a tenolysis such as this, inject up to 30 ml of 1% lidocaine with 1:100,000 epinephrine and up to 3 ml of 8.4% sodium bicarbonate (1 ml of bicarbonate for each 10 ml of 1% lidocaine with 1:100,000 epinephrine).

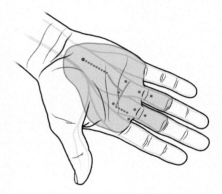

- A 63-year-old woman was unable to flex her long and ring fingers since a tendon repair at age 3 (see the figure above and Clip 38-4). The clip shows injection of local anesthetic, the tenolysis, and the final restored range of motion in the long and ring fingers after 60 years of inability to flex.

- See Chapter 1, Atlas, for more illustrations of the anatomy of diffusion of tumescent local anesthetic in the forearm, wrist, and hand.

SPECIFICS OF MINIMALLY PAINFUL INJECTION OF LOCAL ANESTHETIC IN TENOLYSIS

- Inject the first 10 ml into the most proximal red dot injection point, which is the most proximal incision you are likely to use to dissect the proximal tendon. In this case, we actually injected starting at the wrist crease as we opened the carpal tunnel to make certain it would not be too tight after surgery.

- The first few milliliters of local anesthetic go under the skin, and the rest is injected under the superficial palmar fascia.

- After the common digital nerves of the palm are totally numb (30 minutes is ideal), you can make all of the farther distal epinephrine effect injections in a pain-free manner. Alternatively, you can continue injecting slowly in an antegrade fashion so there is always 1 cm of local anesthetic ahead of the needle, as described in Chapter 5 for minimal pain injection.

- Inject the distal palm with 3 ml in each of the red dots just proximal to the preexisting scar.

- Inject another 2 ml in the subcutaneous fat in each of the three most distal red dots in the palm, which are distal to the scar.

- Note that preexisting scar in the hand creates a natural barrier for diffusion of the local anesthetic. You should start proximally, then inject all around a scar, because the local anesthetic will not traverse it easily, and it is hard to inject into scar.

- Inject another 2 ml in the affected proximal phalanges just under the skin.

- Slowly inject until the whole area you will dissect gets a little firm, with visible and palpable local anesthetic swelling. The goal of the injection is to bathe local anesthetic 2 cm beyond wherever you think you even have a small chance of dissecting. You will not cause a palm compartment syndrome. As soon as you incise the skin, the pressure will come down as the local anesthetic leaks out.

- If you inject 20 ml into the palm, where will it go? Everywhere! Perfect! It is like an extravascular Bier block, but only where you need it, and without a tourniquet.

- We keep the total dose of infiltration less than 7 mg/kg. If less than 50 ml will be required to produce tumescent local anesthesia (see Chapter 4), we use premixed 1% lidocaine with 1:100,000 epinephrine. If 50 to 100 ml is required, we dilute with saline solution to a concentration of 0.5% lidocaine with 1:200,000 epinephrine.

- Inject patients before they come into the operating room, as described in Chapters 3, 4, 5, and 14, to give the lidocaine and epinephrine at least 30 minutes to work.

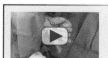

Clip 38-4 Tenolysis in a 63-year-old woman who had been unable to flex her long and ring fingers since a tendon repair at age 3.

IF YOU ARE WORKING WITH AN ANESTHESIOLOGIST

- Ask him or her to use only propofol. Inject the lidocaine with epinephrine as soon as the propofol permits pain-free injection of local anesthetic. This will give the epinephrine a little time to become more effective. The anesthesiologist can then wake the patient right away while you are scrubbing, prepping, and draping so you can get the benefit of intraoperative patient teaching (Chapter 8) and fully cooperative pain-free movement. Suggest that the anesthesia provider avoid administering opiates and amnestics to prevent nausea and permit the patient to remember your intraoperative advice. Patients will also remember the range of motion they can achieve.

TIPS AND TRICKS FOR PERFORMING TENOLYSIS WITH THE WIDE AWAKE APPROACH

Clip 38-5 Patient ruptures her own adhesions in the extensor tendons after wrist fusion.

- Keep testing intraoperative active patient flexion until you get a full range of active motion on the operating table before you close the skin.

- Have the patient pull on the tendons (make a fist) from time to time as you dissect. You will see the patient perform mini-ruptures of adhesions. The patient's movement will guide you to where the tendon is still stuck and where you have to do more dissection to free it.

- We explain to patients during the surgery that we have weakened their tendon by decreasing its blood supply by cutting all of the adhesions. If they use the hand for heavy lifting early after surgery, they could rupture the weakened tendon. They can apply gradual resistance after 14 days when the risk of rupture is less. We treat tenolysed flexor tendons as we treat freshly repaired tendons postoperatively, with gentle early protected movement after passive mobilization of the joint to take out the friction (see Chapter 32).

- We also explain to patients during the surgery that we want them to keep their hand elevated with minimal movement for the first 2 to 4 days to let internal bleeding stop and to allow friction-causing edema to settle. Internal bleeding leads to further internal scarring as the white cells need to "mop up" the old clot. Collagen formation does not start for 3 days. Waiting a few days also allows the avascular tendon to recover from the decrease in blood supply we have caused by cutting adhesions. There is no downside to a rest period, but there are many downsides to immediate forceful movement—especially rupture.

- We do not like to use sedation and amnestics, because many patients may not be able to cooperate as well to pull and rupture their adhesions. They may also not remember the range of active motion they achieved during surgery.

- Many patients are interested in looking at the tendon to understand the nature of their problem. You can mask patients, show them the tendon, and have them watch it move. They will certainly love seeing their stuck tendon move again.

- It is very helpful to have hand therapists attend the tenolysis. They will be able to witness the achievable range of motion and be able to perform intraoperative teaching of the patient along with the surgeon (see Chapter 15).

CHAPTER 39

TENDON TRANSFERS

Donald H. Lalonde, Robert M. Szabo, Mark E. Baratz

ADVANTAGES OF WALANT VERSUS SEDATION AND TOURNIQUET IN TENDON TRANSFERS

- The biggest advantage of using the wide awake approach for tendon transfer is getting the correct tension on the transfer. It is easy to make a tendon transfer too tight or too loose. You can see that your tendon transfer tension is correct by watching the patient take the thumb or finger through a full range of motion before you close the skin.[1] You can tighten or loosen the transfer and have the comfortable, pain-free patient retest the tension. Both you and your patient know the tension is right before you close the skin.

- In Clip 39-2 Dr. Robert Szabo performs a wide awake EI to EPL transfer with intraoperative testing to make sure the tendon transfer is right.

- You can explain to your patient how to activate the transfer during the surgery. Some patients need to think that they are lifting their index finger to get their thumb to move with extensor indicis (EI) to extensor pollicis longus (EPL) tendon transfer. Most patients are able to extend the thumb without initially thinking about lifting the index finger.

- Patients are able to see that their transfer is working during surgery. They are motivated to achieve the result they know they will get if they work at it after surgery.

- In Clip 39-3 Dr. Mark Baratz demonstrates a patient watching herself extend her thumb in the procedure room.

- All of the general advantages listed in Chapter 2 apply to both the surgeon and the patient.

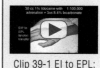

Clip 39-1 EI to EPL: getting the transfer tension right; clinical experience.

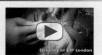

Clip 39-2 Dr. Robert Szabo performs a wide awake EI to EPL transfer.

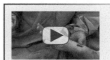

Clip 39-3 Dr. Mark Baratz demonstrates a patient watching herself extend her thumb.

WHERE TO INJECT THE LOCAL ANESTHETIC FOR EI TO EPL TRANSFER

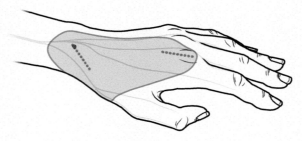

Inject 30 to 40 ml of 1% lidocaine with 1:100,000 epinephrine buffered with 3 to 4 ml of 8.4% bicarbonate (1 ml of sodium bicarbonate for each 10 ml of 1% lidocaine with 1:100,000 epinephrine). The dotted red lines are the possible incisions.

WHERE TO INJECT THE LOCAL ANESTHETIC FOR FLEXOR DIGITORUM SUPERFICIALIS 3 OR 4 (FDS3 OR FDS4) TO THE FLEXOR POLLICIS LONGUS (FPL) TRANSFER

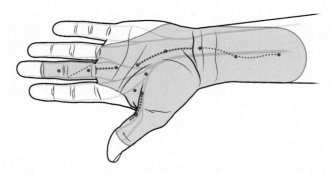

Inject 50 to 100 ml of 0.5% lidocaine with 1:200,000 epinephrine buffered with 10:1 8.4% sodium bicarbonate. Add 10 ml 0.5% bupivacaine with 1:200,000 epinephrine to the total injectate in cases anticipated to last more than 2½ hours, in case the effects of the lidocaine begin to wear off.

- See Chapter 1, Atlas, for more illustrations of the anatomy of diffusion of tumescent local anesthetic in the forearm, wrist, and hand.

SPECIFICS OF INJECTING MINIMALLY PAINFUL LOCAL ANESTHETIC FOR TENDON TRANSFERS

- Inject the anesthetic solution a minimum of 30 minutes before surgery to allow the epinephrine to take optimal effect and provide an adequately dry working field.[2,3]

- We inject supine patients lying down on stretchers in a waiting area to decrease the risk of their fainting (see Chapter 6).

- To minimize the pain of injection, use a 27-gauge needle (not a 25-gauge) into the most proximal injection point (red dot). This point is marked at least 2 cm proximal to the most proximal place you are likely to dissect.

- Ask the patient to look away. Press with a fingertip just proximal to the injection site before you insert the needle to add the sensory "noise" of pressure to decrease the pain. You can also pinch loose forearm skin lightly and push the skin into the needle to decrease pain.

- Insert the first needle perpendicularly into the subcutaneous fat. Stabilize the syringe with two hands and have your thumb ready on the plunger to avoid the pain of needle wobble until the skin needle site is numb. Inject the first visible 0.5 ml bleb and then pause. Wait 15 to 45 seconds until the patient tells you that all the needle pain is gone. Inject the rest of the first 10 ml slowly (over 2 minutes) without moving the needle.

- Continue injecting from proximal to distal, blowing the local anesthetic slowly ahead of the needle so there is always at least 1 cm of visible or palpable local anesthetic ahead of the sharp needle tip that the patient would feel if you advanced it into "live" nerves. "Blow slow before you go." (See Chapter 5 for further tips on how to inject the local anesthetic with minimal pain.)

- Reinsert the needle farther distally into clearly vasoconstricted white skin that has functioning lidocaine and epinephrine so the needle reinsertion is pain free.

- The goal of the injection is to bathe local anesthetic 2 cm beyond wherever you think you even have a small chance of dissecting.

- We keep the total dose of infiltration less than 7 mg/kg. If you need less than 50 ml to produce tumescent local anesthesia (see Chapter 4), use buffered 1% lidocaine with 1:100,000 epinephrine. If you want 50 to 100 ml of volume to inject, dilute with saline solution to a concentration of 0.5% lidocaine with 1:200,000 epinephrine. If you need 100 to 200 ml of volume for larger forearm transfers, dilute buffered 50 ml of commercially available 1% lidocaine with 1:100,000 epinephrine with 150 ml of saline solution to produce 200 ml of 0.25% lidocaine with 1:400,000 epinephrine, which is clinically very effective both for local anesthesia and for vasoconstriction.

- You can inject large areas with blunt-tipped cannulas faster but still pain free. See Chapter 5 for a video clip of cannula injection of tumescent local anesthetic for synovectomy and EI to EPL tendon transfer.

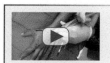

Clip 39-4 How to inject local anesthetic for EI to EPL transfer.

IF YOU ARE WORKING WITH AN ANESTHESIOLOGIST

- Ask him or her to use only propofol. Inject the lidocaine with epinephrine as soon as the propofol permits pain-free injection of local anesthetic. This will give the epinephrine a little time to become more effective. The anesthesiologist can then wake the patient right away while you are scrubbing, prepping, and draping so you can get the benefit of intraoperative patient teaching (Chapter 8) and fully cooperative pain-free movement. Suggest that the anesthesia provider avoid administering opiates and amnestics to prevent nausea and permit the patient to remember your intraoperative advice. Patients will also remember the range of motion they can achieve.

TIPS AND TRICKS FOR PERFORMING TENDON TRANSFERS WITH THE WIDE AWAKE APPROACH

- What you see on the table with intraoperative transfer tension testing is what you will get as a result. If the transfer looks too loose, it will be too loose postoperatively. If it looks too tight, it will be too tight postoperatively.

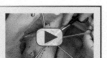

Clip 39-5 EI to EPL surgery with intraoperative testing of thumb flexion and extension.

- Do not be afraid to test full flexion and full extension. Your sutures should be strong enough to take it. If they are not, you need to reinforce them.

- Patients may need to look at their fingers or thumb when you ask them to test the transfer, since they may not feel the numbed digits. Although most patients do not mind looking at the wound, you can cover the wound with a towel as they watch their fingers and thumb move.

Clip 39-6 Another video of EI to EPL surgery with intraoperative testing of thumb flexion and extension.

- Many patients are interested in looking at the tendon to understand the nature of their problem. You can mask them, show them the tendon, and have them watch it move. It will help greatly that they see the transfer move, because they know that it will work after they overcome the pain and stiffness.

- If you want the thumb EPL to relax, ask the patient to flex the thumb IP joint. The spinal cord reflex will force the EPL to relax.[4]

- If you are going to remove a radius fracture volar plate at the same time you are performing an FDS to FPL tendon transfer, you will need more local anesthetic. In the case shown in Clip 39-7, we used 125 ml of 0.25% lidocaine with 1:400,000 epinephrine and added 10 ml 0.5% bupivacaine with 1:200,000 epinephrine, because we knew the case might take longer than 2½ hours. We injected the local anesthetic down onto the plate and the bone diffusely on both sides of the radius where the plate was located.

Clip 39-7 FDS4 to FPL transfer with radius plate removal.

- We have patients relieve themselves in the restroom after we inject the local anesthetic and just before we start the surgery to avoid unnecessary surgical interruptions for these longer cases. Patients do not receive an intravenous fluid that increases the urge to void. If we give preoperative antibiotics, we give them by mouth.

- For older patients with cardiac comorbidities, you can decrease the concentration of epinephrine and perform the WALANT procedure in the hospital main operating room with monitoring.

- In Clip 39-8, an 84-year-old man with cardiac issues was given a lowered epinephrine concentration in the hospital and was monitored during WALANT surgery for EI to EPL tendon transfer.

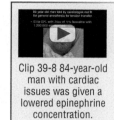

Clip 39-8 84-year-old man with cardiac issues was given a lowered epinephrine concentration.

References

1. Lalonde D. Wide-awake extensor indicis proprius to extensor pollicis longus tendon transfer. J Hand Surg 39:2297, 2014.
2. Lalonde DH, Wong A. Dosage of local anesthesia in wide awake hand surgery. J Hand Surg Am 38:2025, 2013.
3. McKee DE, Lalonde DH, Thoma A, Glennie DL, Hayward JE. Optimal time delay between epinephrine injection and incision to minimize bleeding. Plast Reconstr Surg 131:811, 2013.
4. Bezuhly M, Sparkes GL, Higgins A, Neumeister M, Lalonde DH. Immediate thumb extension following extensor indicis proprius to extensor pollicis longus tendon transfer using the wide-awake approach. Plast Reconstr Surg 119:1507, 2007.

CHAPTER 40
LACERATED NERVES

Donald H. Lalonde

ADVANTAGES OF WALANT VERSUS SEDATION AND TOURNIQUET IN REPAIR OF LACERATED NERVES

- You are able to see how much tension there is on your nerve repair with the patient's active movement before you close the skin. You may decide to let the patient go back to work 3 to 7 days postoperatively with a relative motion flexion splint (see the relative motion flexion splint in Clip 40-1 and other videos in Chapters 35 and 36).

- During surgery you will have the unhurried time to explain to the patient all of the problems of a nerve laceration. You can explain in simple terms what to expect over the next few months, including his or her ability to return to work and the best way to take pain medications after surgery. Your patient can remember and absorb all of this in a pain-free, unsedated state.

- All of the general advantages listed in Chapter 2 apply to both the surgeon and the patient.

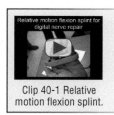

Clip 40-1 Relative motion flexion splint.

WHERE TO INJECT THE LOCAL ANESTHETIC FOR REPAIR OF DIGITAL NERVE LACERATIONS

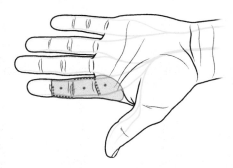

The orange line in the illustration is the laceration and the dotted red lines are the possible incisions. Inject 8 ml of 1% lidocaine with 1:100,000 epinephrine (buffered with 10 ml lido/epi:1 ml of 8.4% sodium bicarbonate).

- See Chapter 1, Atlas, for more illustrations of the anatomy of diffusion of tumescent local anesthetic in the forearm, wrist, and hand.

SPECIFICS OF MINIMALLY PAINFUL INJECTION OF LOCAL ANESTHETIC FOR REPAIR OF LACERATED NERVES

- Inject the anesthetic solution a minimum of 30 minutes before surgery to allow the lidocaine and epinephrine to take optimal effect and provide an adequately dry working field, as outlined in Chapters 3, 4, and 14. Inject the patient in the waiting area outside the procedure room so no time is wasted.

- We inject supine patients lying down on stretchers to decrease the risk of their fainting (Chapter 6).

- To minimize the pain of injection, inject with a fine 27-gauge needle (not a 25-gauge).

- Ask the patient to look away. Press with a fingertip just proximal to the injection site before you put in the needle to add the sensory "noise" of pressure to decrease the pain.

- Insert the first needle perpendicularly into the subcutaneous fat. Stabilize the syringe with two hands and have your thumb ready on the plunger to avoid the pain of needle wobble until the skin needle site is numb. Inject the first visible 0.5 ml bleb and then pause. Wait 15 to 45 seconds until your patient tells you that all the needle pain is gone. Inject the rest of the first 4 ml slowly (over 2 minutes) without moving the needle.

- Inject the first 4 ml of 1% lidocaine with 1:100,000 epinephrine buffered 10:1 with 8.4% sodium bicarbonate in the most proximal injection point in the distal palm.

- Ideally, wait 30 minutes to let the digital nerves get numb so the next injections will be pain free. Then inject 2 ml subcutaneously in each of the injection points in the subcutaneous fat in the center of the proximal and middle phalanges.

WHERE TO INJECT THE LOCAL ANESTHETIC FOR REPAIR OF A MEDIAN NERVE LACERATION IN THE FOREARM

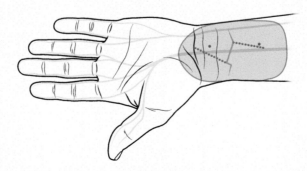

Inject 30 to 50 ml of 1% lidocaine with 1:100,000 epinephrine (buffered with 10 ml lido/epi:1 ml of 8.4% sodium bicarbonate).

- See Chapter 1, Atlas, for more illustrations of the anatomy of diffusion of tumescent local anesthetic in the forearm, wrist, and hand.

SPECIFICS OF INJECTING THE LOCAL ANESTHETIC FOR REPAIR OF A MEDIAN NERVE LACERATION IN THE FOREARM

- Inject patients before they come into the procedure room, as outlined in Chapters 3, 4, 5, and 14, to give the local anesthetic at least 45 to 60 minutes to work for major nerve lacerations such as the median nerve.

- Always start by injecting well proximal to the laceration where the nerve is "live" to anesthetize the nerve. You can inject distal to the laceration after the entire area proximal to the laceration is completely numb.

- Inject 25 ml of 1% lidocaine with 1:100,000 epinephrine buffered 10:1 with 8.4% sodium bicarbonate 2 to 3 cm proximal to the laceration. The first 15 ml is injected just under the skin and the remaining 10 ml is placed subfascially.

- Gradually advance the needle as you inject the 25 ml, as described in Chapter 5, for minimal pain injection. The fascia is 3 to 5 mm under the skin, depending on the patient's size. It is best to have extra local anesthetic at hand, because some of it may well come out through the laceration.

- We keep the total dose of infiltration less than 7 mg/kg. If less than 50 ml will be required to produce tumescent local anesthesia (see Chapter 4), we use premixed 1% lidocaine with 1:100,000 epinephrine. If 50 to 100 ml is required, we dilute with saline solution to a concentration of 0.5% lidocaine with 1:200,000 epinephrine.

- Consider adding 10 ml of 0.5% bupivacaine with 1:200,000 epinephrine or liposomal bupivacaine to produce longer pain relief for major nerve lacerations.

- Inject another 10 to 15 ml of local anesthetic to tumesce the skin distal to the laceration.

- Be sure to have at least 5 cm of visible palpable local anesthetic proximal to the laceration along the path of the nerve.

TIPS AND TRICKS FOR REPAIRING LACERATED NERVES WITH THE WIDE AWAKE APPROACH

- We have performed a level I evidence study (still to be published) that shows that large nerve blocks such as in the median nerve increase in intensity over 90 minutes after injection. We therefore inject patients and have them wait an hour or more if possible for the nerve to become completely numb while we see other patients or operate in the clinic. In this way, no time is wasted and the patient with lacerated nerves experiences no pain during the repair.

- If you cannot wait for 60 minutes for a median or ulnar nerve to get numb, you can approach the "live nerve" very carefully at surgery. Expose it above the laceration. Inject the loose areolar tissue outside the healthy proximal part of the nerve with a 30-gauge needle with the bevel parallel to the nerve. This will balloon the outside covering of the nerve to accelerate nerve infiltration by the lidocaine. Do not inject inside the nerve perineurium or elicit paresthesias, because you may damage axons.

- For digital nerve injuries, you can simulate relative motion flexion splinting for early protected movement to begin 3 to 5 days after surgery. Repair the nerve and insert a tongue depressor, as in Clip 40-1.

- If the nerve stays together with no tension with active flexion and extension, you can prescribe a relative motion flexion splint to be worn postoperatively. If the nerve comes apart with tongue depressor simulation, then clearly you would treat this patient with standard immobilization after surgery.

- We perform these nerve repairs in the clinic with field sterility (see Chapter 10) and loupe magnification.

CHAPTER 41
FINGER FRACTURES

Donald H. Lalonde

ADVANTAGES OF WALANT VERSUS SEDATION AND TOURNIQUET FOR FINGER FRACTURE REDUCTION

- When you see full flexion and extension of the finger you have K-wired at surgery and see that your reduction is stable with fluoroscopy, you will feel a lot more comfortable about starting early protected movement for these fingers, just as in flexor tendon injuries.[1,2]

- After you reduce the fractures, you can watch the patient, who is comforable and tourniquet free, move the reconstructed bone to see how stable the fixation is. You can add more K-wires if you feel greater stability is needed to support early protected movement.

- You can see whether the K-wires are interrupting active finger movement by impinging on ligaments or tendons in their current location. You have the opportunity to change the K-wire location to optimize postoperative early active movement before the end of the operation.

- A major advantage of eliminating sedation for finger fractures is that you do not need to perform the reduction in the main operating room (see Chapters 10 and 16). If patients need internal fixation, you can perform closed reduction and K-wire insertion in minor procedure rooms in the clinic outside the main operating room Monday to Friday, 9 AM to 5 PM (see Clip 41-3). You no longer need to do these at night to suit the main operating room and anesthesiologist's schedules. You are more likely to do better surgery with a clear head at 1 PM than when you are tired at 1 AM. You no longer have to admit patients to the hospital because of their medical comorbidities; these issues are only a problem when you use sedation.

- Because you can perform these operations in the clinic, your hand therapists can see how much active finger movement is possible during the surgery. You can discuss the safe early protected movement plan with therapists during and after the surgery (see Chapter 15).

- All of the general advantages listed in Chapter 2 apply to both the surgeon and the patient.

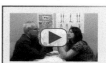

Clip 41-1 Early protected movement 3 days after K-wiring middle phalanx fracture.

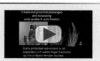

Clip 41-2 Two finger fractures: numbing, intraoperative testing of functionally stable fixation of K-wire reduction, early protected movement demonstration, and final result.

Clip 41-3 Augmented field sterility setup for inserting K-wires in a minor procedure room.

WHERE TO INJECT THE LOCAL ANESTHETIC FOR FINGER FRACTURE REDUCTION

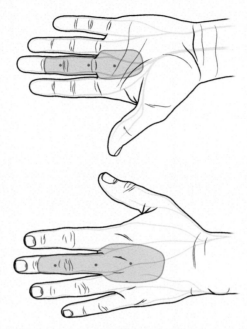

Palmar injections: Inject 4 ml of 1% lidocaine with 1:100,000 epinephrine (buffered with 10 ml lido/epi:1 ml of 8.4% sodium bicarbonate) in the most proximal red injection point on the palmar side. Do the most proximal dorsal injection next, and then inject 2 ml in the middle of each of the palmar proximal and middle phalanges in the subcutaneous fat. *Dorsal injections:* Inject 4 ml of 1% lidocaine with 1:100,000 epinephrine (buffered with 10 ml lido/epi:1 ml of 8.4% sodium bicarbonate) bicarbonate in the proximal red injection dot on the dorsal hand. Do the two palmar injections next, and then inject 2 ml in the middle of each of the dorsal proximal and middle phalanges in the subcutaneous fat.

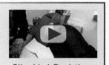

Clip 41-4 Real-time minimal pain local injection for proximal phalanx fracture.

- See Chapter 1, Atlas, for more illustrations of the anatomy of diffusion of tumescent local anesthetic in the forearm, wrist, and hand.

SPECIFICS OF MINIMALLY PAINFUL INJECTION OF LOCAL ANESTHETIC FOR FINGER FRACTURE REDUCTION

- Inject just under the skin. There is no need to inject into the sheath; this would only add unnecessary pain. The local anesthetic will diffuse into the sheath.

- Inject the anesthetic solution a minimum of 30 minutes before surgery to allow the epinephrine to take optimal effect and provide an adequately dry working field,[3] as outlined in Chapters 4 and 14.

- Inject patients in a waiting area before they come into the procedure room to give the local anesthetic time to work.

- We inject supine patients lying down on stretchers to decrease the risk of their fainting (see Chapter 6).

- To minimize the pain of injection, inject with a 27-gauge needle (not a 25-gauge).

- Ask the patient to look away. Press with a fingertip just proximal to the injection site before you put in the needle to add the sensory "noise" of pressure to decrease the pain. (See Chapter 5 for other hints on how to decrease the pain of local injection.)

- Start with the first 4 ml in the proximal palmar red injection point. Then inject 4 ml just under the skin on the dorsal side's most proximal red dot injection point.

- Insert the first needle perpendicularly into the subcutaneous fat. Stabilize the syringe with two hands and have the thumb ready on the plunger to avoid the pain of needle wobble until the skin needle site is numb. Inject the first visible 0.5 ml bleb and then pause. Wait 15 to 45 seconds until the patient tells you that all the needle pain is gone. Inject the rest of the 4 ml slowly (over 1 to 2 minutes) without moving the needle.

- There is no need to move the needle, since the local anesthetic will diffuse through the fat, unless there is previous scarring.

- If convenient, wait 15 to 30 minutes before injecting distally on the palmar side and dorsal sides so the next two digital palmar and dorsal injections will not be painful. This waiting period can be used productively to see other patients.

- Follow with the next pain-free injections. Inject 2 ml just under the skin on the palmar side in the red injection points of the proximal and middle phalanges. Then inject 2 ml just under the skin on the dorsal side in the red injection points of the proximal and middle phalanges.

- It is worth injecting into the middle phalanx if you are operating on a proximal phalanx fracture, because the epinephrine will help with hemostasis and decrease internal bleeding, which would occupy space and be replaced with inflammatory tissue.

- There is no need to inject into the distal phalanx dorsum, since bleeding will be minimal if you have injected in the dorsal middle phalanx.

- If you are only using K-wires for a percutaneous reduction and not cutting through the skin, it is still worth having epinephrine in the soft tissue around the bone you are K-wiring, even if that tissue is numb from proximal blocks. Epinephrine will provide less internal bleeding in the periosteal tissue, which means less callus and less scar for the patient to work through later.

TIPS AND TRICKS FOR PERFORMING FINGER FRACTURE REDUCTION WITH THE WIDE AWAKE APPROACH

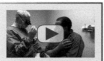

Clip 41-5 Advice to an awake patient at the end of finger fracture reduction surgery.

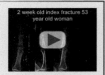

Clip 41-6 Testing stability of dorsal blocking K-wire for dorsal fracture dislocation of PIP joint.

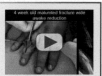

Clip 41-7 Wide awake operative reduction of a 4-week-old scissoring malunion of the proximal phalanx.

- Patients may need to look at their fingers or thumb to help them move the digit after you reduce the fracture, since they cannot feel the numbed digit move. Although most patients do not mind looking at the wound, you can cover it with a towel as they flex and extend the tip of the finger or thumb.

- Take advantage of the fact that the patient is not sedated to give him or her clear instructions on postoperative activity. You can get better patient cooperation for postoperative hand elevation and care because the patient is able to listen and remember your advice right at the end of surgery. This can decrease your complication risk.

- Clip 41-5 shows advice to an awake patient at the end of finger fracture reduction surgery. (See Chapter 8 for other videos on intraoperative advice for patients.)

- An experienced surgeon can insert a K-wire quickly and safely with field sterility. If the K-wiring will take a long time because it is difficult, or if we may need to open the skin to reduce the fracture, we import gowns and half sheets to the clinic for augmented field sterility (see Clip 41-3). There is no rule that says that an added gown and half sheet sterility are restricted to the main operating room.

- You can test the stability of your dorsal blocking K-wire when using this technique for dorsal fracture dislocations of the PIP joint for early protected movement (see Clip 41-6).

- You can test the stability of your internal fixation and the active mobility of the tendons and joints intraoperatively in complex malunion reduction cases (see Clip 41-7).

- For comminuted intraarticular PIP and MP fractures that require distraction splinting, consider inserting K-wires for distraction splinting in the clinic. We have the therapists apply a banjo distraction splint while the patient's hand is still numb. You can then assess the joint in the splint with fluoroscopy while the patient is still numb, as in Clip 41-8. You can change the K-wire while the patient's hand is still numb if necessary.

- Some finger fractures don't need surgery (see Clip 41-9).

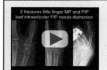

Clip 41-8 Distraction splint for comminuted PIP and MP fractures.

References

1. Gregory S, Lalonde DH, Leung LT. Minimally invasive finger fracture management, wide-awake closed reduction, K-wire fixation, and early protective movement. In Curtin C, Chung KC, eds. Hand Clinics: Minimally Invasive Hand Surgery. London: Elsevier, 2014.
2. Jones NF, Jupiter JB, Lalonde DH. Common fractures and dislocations of the hand. Plast Reconstr Surg 130:722e, 2012.
3. McKee DE, Lalonde DH, Thoma A, Glennie DL, Hayward JE. Optimal time delay between epinephrine injection and incision to minimize bleeding. Plast Reconstr Surg 131:811, 2013.

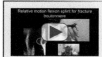

Clip 41-9 Fracture boutonniere treated with a relative motion flexion splint only.

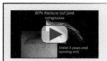

Clip 41-10 Mallet fractures involving 50% to 60% of the joint but with congruous or parallel joint surfaces (not subluxated) can be treated with mallet splinting only.

CHAPTER 42
REDUCTION AND INTERNAL FIXATION OF METACARPAL FRACTURES

Shu Guo Xing, Jin Bo Tang, Donald H. Lalonde

ADVANTAGES OF WALANT VERSUS SEDATION AND TOURNIQUET IN REDUCTION AND INTERNAL FIXATION OF METACARPAL FRACTURES

- You can see that you have solved the scissoring problem by watching your patient take the fingers through a full range of active motion before you close the skin.

- Patients see the reduction of their bone on fluoroscopy. They watch themselves achieve a full range of flexion and extension of their fingers during the surgery. They remember this and know that this will be achievable if they stick with therapy and exercise after the surgery.

- You and your hand therapist can educate wide awake patients during the operation to instill the importance of postoperative therapy into patients' consciousness.

- Patients can practice postoperative movement in a pain-free state during surgery.

- You can check the stability of the bone fixation with full flexion and extension during the surgery. This helps you to decide whether or not to allow early protected movement after surgery.

- All of the general advantages listed in Chapter 2 apply to both the surgeon and the patient.

WHERE TO INJECT THE LOCAL ANESTHETIC FOR REDUCTION AND INTERNAL FIXATION OF METACARPAL FRACTURES

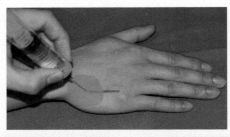

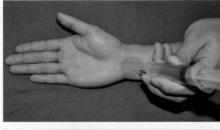
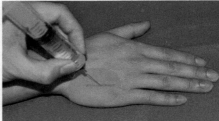

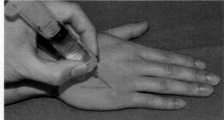
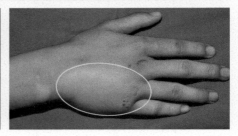

Inject a total of 30 to 40 ml of 1% lidocaine with 1:100,000 epinephrine (buffered with 10 ml lido/epi:1 ml of 8.4% sodium bicarbonate).

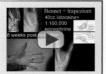

Clip 42-1 Fracture dislocation at the base of the thumb metacarpal (Bennett fracture).

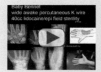

Clip 42-2 Fracture dislocation at the base of the fifth metacarpal.

- See Chapter 1, Atlas, for illustrations of the anatomy of diffusion of tumescent local anesthetic in the forearm, wrist, and hand.

- Local anesthesia for a Bennett fracture is the same as for a trapeziectomy (see Chapter 27). You flood the radial side of the hand with 40 ml of buffered lidocaine with epinephrine, as shown in Clip 42-1.

- The local anesthetic for fracture dislocations of the fourth and fifth metacarpal bases is 40 ml of buffered lidocaine and epinephrine flooding the ulnar side of the distal wrist and base of the hand, as shown in Clip 42-2.

SPECIFICS OF MINIMALLY PAINFUL INJECTION OF LOCAL ANESTHETIC IN REDUCTION AND INTERNAL FIXATION OF METACARPAL FRACTURES

- To minimize the pain of injection, inject with a 27-gauge needle (not a 25-gauge).

- The first 10 ml goes into the most proximal location that you will dissect.

- Ask the patient to look away. Press with a fingertip just proximal to the injection site before you put in the needle to add the sensory "noise" of pressure to decrease the pain.

- Insert the first needle perpendicularly into the subcutaneous fat. Stabilize the syringe with two hands to avoid the pain of needle wobble until the skin needle site is numb. Inject the first visible 0.5 ml bleb and then pause. Wait 15 to 45 seconds until the patient tells you that all the needle pain is gone. Inject the rest of the first 10 ml slowly (over 2 to 3 minutes) without moving the needle (see Chapter 5).

- You may inject an additional 10 ml between the median and ulnar nerves under the forearm fascia at the volar wrist if you would like to block those nerves with tumescent local anesthetic.

- Inject the second 10 ml of local anesthetic in the center of the incision site with the needle inserted into clearly vasoconstricted white skin that has functioning lidocaine and epinephrine so that needle insertion is pain free. You should have tumescent local anesthetic (Chapter 4) diffused at least 2 cm on either side of the incision.

- Inject the third 10 ml in the distal third of the incision.

- The goal of the injection is to bathe local anesthetic all around the metacarpal where dissection or internal fixation will occur, including the palmar side and between the metacarpals. You may want to add additional local anesthetic in the lateral and volar aspects of the metacarpal with a fourth 10 ml syringe.

- Inject the anesthetic solution in a waiting area a minimum of 30 minutes before surgery to allow the epinephrine to take optimal effect and provide an adequately dry working field. This waiting period can be used productively to see other patients.

- We inject supine patients lying down on stretchers to decrease the risk of their fainting (see Chapter 6).

- For articular fractures, add 2 to 4 ml into the joint cavity and in the soft tissues around the joint.

- For plate removal, bathe the entire surgical dissection area with ample local anesthetic from proximal to distal on both sides of the surgical scar. Let the local anesthetic diffuse into the scar on its own. You should have 2 cm of local anesthetic all around the planned dissection area (see Clip 42-4).

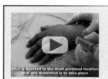

Clip 42-3 Local anesthesia for fourth and fifth metacarpal operative reduction.

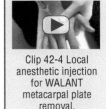

Clip 42-4 Local anesthetic injection for WALANT metacarpal plate removal.

TIPS AND TRICKS FOR PERFORMING REDUCTION AND INTERNAL FIXATION OF METACARPAL FRACTURES WITH THE WIDE AWAKE APPROACH

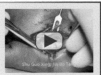

Clip 42-5 Operative reduction of fourth and fifth metacarpal fractures in the patient injected with local anesthetic seen in Clip 42-3.

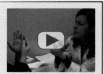

Clip 42-6 Early protected movement 3 days after K-wire fixation of a metacarpal fracture.

Clip 42-7 A 3-month-old malunion of a metacarpal with intraoperative testing of full flexion and extension after reduction and plating.

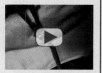

Clip 42-8 Checking scissoring after dynamic compression bone clamp metacarpal fracture reduction.

• After you have provisional reduction, ask the patient to make a fist and extend the fingers to test the stability of your internal fixation. You will see whether there is enough stability in the fixation to support early protected movement or whether you need to insert additional fixation.

• You can correct any malrotation that the patient demonstrates with intraoperative active flexion and extension before you close the skin.

• A dynamic compression bone clamp provides enough temporary rigid fixation in transverse metacarpal fractures that you can test full flexion and full extension of the clamp-held reduced fractures to make sure there is no malrotation before you drill screw holes.

Part IV

COMPLEX RECONSTRUCTIONS

CHAPTER 43

COMPLEX RECONSTRUCTIONS IN HAND SURGERY

Donald H. Lalonde, Jason Wong, Alistair Phillips, Nik Jagodzinski

Many complex reconstructions are undertaken when movement after trauma or surgery does not produce ideal function. The goal is usually to restore useful movement of the wrist, thumb, and fingers. Patients with sedation, a motor block, or a tourniquet are not able to move reconstructed parts during surgery in comfort. WALANT permits them to do just that. Furthermore, the surgeon can adjust the reconstruction to make it work if the preoperative plan is successful when patients move reconstructed fingers or thumbs during the surgery. The more complex the reconstruction, the more helpful WALANT can be. We present a video series of cases to illustrate this point.

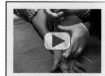

Clip 43-1 Repair of a 5½-week-old FPL laceration.

- Clip 43-1 shows a repair of a 5½-week-old flexor pollicis longus (FPL) laceration. We did not know which operation would be possible or best—primary repair, primary palmaris longus tendon graft, or tendon transfer of the long finger flexor digitorum superficialis (FDS). We injected local anesthetic for all three possibilities and made our decision based on active movement by the patient during the surgery.

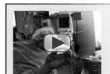

Clip 43-2 Change thumb tip pinch after adult pollicization.

- Clip 43-2 demonstrates a change in thumb tip pinch after adult pollicization. This patient had an adult pollicization of the index finger after a failed thumb replantation. Years later, he requested better thumb tip pinch and was able to participate in selecting the perfect angle during the surgery.

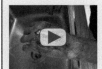

Clip 43-3 Cleaning a severely contaminated hand wound in the emergency department.

- Clip 43-3 describes cleaning a severely contaminated hand wound in the emergency department. This illustrates how we wash very contaminated wounds with tap water after adequate local anesthetic is administered in the emergency department.

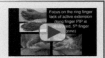

Clip 43-4 Extensor tendon graft of the dorsum of the hand.

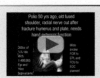

Clip 43-5 FCR and FCU transfer in a polio case.

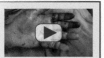

Clip 43-6 Finger revascularization with wrist vein grafts by Dr. Jason Wong.

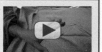

Clip 43-7 Homodigital island flap by Dr. Jason Wong.

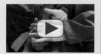

Clip 43-8 Restoration of thumb extension after subtotal amputation.

- Clip 43-4 shows a complex secondary reconstruction with extensor tendon grafting where intraoperative active movement demonstrated that the preoperative plan of simple tendon graft insertion failed because it did not extend the proximal phalanx adequately. We added graft suturing to the proximal extensor hood of the proximal phalanx to the preoperative plan because of intraoperative active extension observation and were ultimately successful.

- Clip 43-5 is of a complex extensor tendon transfer case. The patient had had polio 50 years earlier, which resulted in muscle dysfunction of the entire upper limb and shoulder fusion. She subsequently fractured her humerus and acquired a postplating radial nerve palsy. We planned a flexor carpi radialis (FCR) and flexor carpi ulnaris (FCU) transfer procedure. We saw the true active excursion of the polio affected muscles at surgery that altered the preoperative plan with ultimate success.

- Clip 43-6 shows a finger revascularization with wrist vein grafts by Dr. Jason Wong. The patient had sustained a severe crush injury to all four digits of the left hand, with delayed presentation that rendered the index and middle fingers nonsalvageable. The ring and little fingers were salvaged using the WALANT technique.

- In Clip 43-7 a homodigital island flap was performed by Dr. Jason Wong. This was a case of fingertip reconstruction with a local pedicled island flap with WALANT anesthesia. Active movement during surgery shows correct tension of the inserted pedicle.

- In Clip 43-8 thumb extension was restored after a subtotal amputation. This subtotal amputation of a thumb ended up without extensor pollicis longus (EPL) function. We injected enough local anesthetic to allow extensor indicis proprius (EIP) tendon transfer if the EPL muscle had been too short to permit simple tendon repair.

- Clip 43-9 shows a WALANT FPL repair under the motor branch in the carpal tunnel. The patient ruptured the repair. We also show the secondary repair with WALANT 8 days after the initial repair. Postoperative management of both operations is explained.

- Clip 43-10 shows a swan neck flexor digitorum superficialis (FDS) transfer. We sutured the proximal FDS of the small finger to the proximal phalanx with a bone anchor to correct a swan neck deformity. Active movement during the surgery shows the correct selection of tension.

- In Clip 43-11 a woman in her late sixties presented with rupture of the fourth and fifth extensors of her left hand. We harvested a palmaris longus tendon graft and hooked it up to proximal tendon stump motors that still had good active excursion. We strengthened the repair with a transfer to the long finger extensor and performed a tenodesis of the extensor digiti minimi, all decisions based on active movement at the time of surgery.

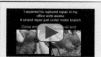

Clip 43-9 Ruptured FPL repair under the motor branch in the carpal tunnel.

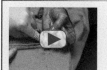

Clip 43-10 Swan neck FDS transfer.

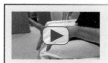

Clip 43-11 Palmaris longus tendon graft for rupture of fourth and fifth extensors.

CONCLUSION

We have found that secondary reconstructions of the hand and fingers in awake pain-free patients have the great benefit of adding voluntary active movement during the surgery. We have often been pleasantly surprised, as we have been in the cases presented here, that outcomes have been improved because of intraoperative adjustments on reconstructed parts based on what we see with patients moving. It has become our method of choice where the goal of the operation is to improve active function.

INDEX

A

Abductor pollicis longus, ligament reconstruction and tendon interposition with, 167
Accountable Care Act (ACA), 96
Accountable care organizations (ACOs), 96
Administrators, 79-80, 91, 112
Airway, 89
Amadio, Peter, 92-94
American Association for Accreditation of Ambulatory Surgery Facilities (AAASF), 76, 118
Amputation
  finger; see Finger amputation
  ray; see Ray amputation
  thumb, extension restoration after, 250
Anesthesia; see General anesthesia; Local anesthesia; Local anesthetics
Anesthesiologists
  barriers to WALANT by, 88-89
  carpal tunnel decompression/release participation by, 135
  description of, 31
  extensor tendon repair participation by
    finger, 211
    forearm, 219
    hand, 215
  flexor tendon repair participation by
    finger, 192
    forearm, 207
    hand, 202
  median nerve release at elbow participation by, 143
  open triangular fibrocartilage complex repair participation by, 185
  proximal interphalangeal joint procedures
    arthroplasty, 163
    fusion, 176
  tendon transfer participation by, 230
  tenolysis participation by, 224
  thumb metacarpophalangeal joint fusion participation by, 173
  trapeziectomy participation by, 168
  ulnar collateral ligament repair participation by, 173
  WALANT buy-in by, 79-81
  working with, 104
  wrist arthroscopy participation by, 182
Anticoagulants, 19-20, 94
Anxious patients, 52, 55
Arthroscopy, wrist; see Wrist arthroscopy

B

Baratz, Mark, 227
Barriers
  anesthesiologist-perceived, 88-89
  general types of, 82-84
  nurse-perceived, 85-86
  patient-perceived, 84-85
  surgeon-perceived, 86-88
Bennett fracture, 244
Blunt cannulas, for local anesthetic injection, 45-46, 218, 229
Bone reconstruction, 56
Boutonniere surgery, 209
Brachial artery, 144
Brazil, 33
Buffering of lidocaine with 1:100,000 epinephrine, with 10:1 8.4% sodium bicarbonate, 37-38, 138
Bupivacaine, 32, 50-51, 100, 230, 235
Buy-in
  from administrators, 79-80
  from anesthesiologists, 79-81
  from nurses, 79-81
  from payers, 79-82

C

Canadian Association for Accreditation of Ambulatory Surgical Facilities (CAAASF), 76, 117
Cannulas, blunt, 45-46, 218

Carpal tunnel decompression/release
    anesthesiologist involvement in, 135
    cubital tunnel decompression and, 140
    endoscopic
        local anesthetic injection for, 133
        tips for, 136
    field sterility versus full sterility for,
        69-71, 134
    local anesthetic injections for, 43, 130-
        133
    open
        local anesthetic injection for, 130-
            132
        tips for, 134-135
    patient education about, 62-63
    patient positioning for, 132
    surgical instrument for, 119
    WALANT benefits for, 21, 129-130
    wound care after, 62
Caseload, 107-108, 129
Catech-o-methyl transferase, 51
Cautery, 105
Cautery machine, 120
Children, 65-67
Comminuted fractures, 241
Complex reconstruction, 249-250
Consultation
    from emergency department, 109
    talking with patient during, 55-57
    from trauma surgery, 109
Cost reductions
    for governments, 78
    for hospitals, 77-78
    for insurance companies, 78
    for operating facility, 77-78
    for patients, 75-76
    for payers, 78
    for surgeons, 76, 96
Creases, skin, 34, 44
Cubital tunnel decompression
    carpal tunnel decompression/release
        and, 140
    description of, 17
    field sterility for, 140
    local anesthetic injection for, 138-139
    patient positioning for, 137, 139-140
    tips for, 139-140
    WALANT advantages for, 137

D
Dalhousie Project experimental phase, 26
De Quervain release, 149-150
Denkler, Keith, 24

Dermis, injection of 0.5 ml with perpen-
    dicular needle just under, 40-41
Dermofasciectomy, 153-154
Desmarres retractors, 119, 148
Difficult surgeries, 87
Digital extension-flexion test, 195
Digital nerve laceration, 233
Dorsal block augmentation, finger block
    with, 12
Dorsal thumb proximal phalanx block, 13
Draping, 85
Driving, 58
Dupuytren's contracture
    local anesthetic injection for, 152-153
    recurrent, 151, 153
    tips for, 153-154
    WALANT advantages for, 151
Dynamic compression bone clamp, 246

E
Education
    of patients, 59-60
    of trainees, 61
Egypt, 33
Emergency department consultations,
    109
Endoscopy
    carpal tunnel decompression/release
        local anesthetic injection for, 133
        tips for, 136
    cubital tunnel decompression, 139
Epinephrine; see also Lidocaine with epi-
    nephrine
    1:1000
        accidental injection of, in finger, 27
        illustration of, 33
        vasoconstriction duration with, 32
    1:10,000, 32
    1:100,000
        definition of, 33
        lidocaine with; see Lidocaine (1%)
            with 1:100,000 epinephrine
        vasoconstriction with, 30, 32
    1:200,000
        definition of, 33
        lidocaine (0.5%) with, 132, 138,
            228, 230
    1:400,000, 121
    1:1,000,000
        clinical uses of, 33
        hemostasis with, 105
    adverse reactions to, 50-51
    author's reasons for using, 24

cardiac responses to, 83, 231
concentrations of, 33
in fingers, 23-24, 83
half-life of, 51
hemostasis uses of, 20, 23-24, 50, 105
history of, 23-24
in hypertensive patients, 50
myths regarding, 24-25
phentolamine reversal of, 24-27, 50, 83
"rush" caused by, 51
safety of, 17, 49-50, 83
vasoconstriction from, 32, 108, 128
Europe, 33
Evidence-based medicine, 78
Extension-flexion test
    after extensor tendon repair of hand, 215
    after flexor tendon repair
        of finger, 195
        of hand, 202
Extensor indicis to extensor pollicis longus tendon transfer, 227-228
Extensor tendon grafting, 250
Extensor tendon repair
    of finger
        anesthesiologist participation in, 211
        local anesthetic injection for, 210-211
        patient education during, 212
        tips for, 211-212
        WALANT advantages for, 209
    of forearm
        anesthesiologist participation in, 219
        incisions for, 217
        local anesthetic injection for, 217-218
        tips for, 219
        WALANT advantages for, 217
    of hand
        anesthesiologist participation in, 215
        extension-flexion testing after, 215
        field sterility for, 216
        local anesthetic injection for, 214-215
        tips for, 215-216
        WALANT advantages for, 213
    hand therapy in, 114
    percutaneous, 211

F
Facilities, local anesthetic injections in, 83-84
Fainting, 51-52, 57
Field sterility
    benefits of, 77
    for carpal tunnel decompression/release, 134
    components of, 95
    for cubital tunnel decompression, 140
    definition of, 69
    for extensor tendon repair of hand, 216
    full sterility versus, 69-72, 77
    in minor procedure rooms, 119
    outcomes with, 71
Fielding, John, 23
Fifteen cases per day, scheduling of, 107-108, 129
Finger
    extensor tendon repair of; see Extensor tendon repair, of finger
    flexor tendon repair of; see Flexor tendon repair, of finger
    infarction of, 27
    revascularization of, with wrist vein grafts, 250
Finger amputation
    local anesthetic injection for, 125-128
    tips and tricks for, 128
    WALANT advantages for, 125
Finger block
    with dorsal block augmentation, 12
    subcutaneous midline proximal phalanx, 11
Finger fracture reduction
    comminuted fractures, 241
    hand therapy after, 114-115
    K-wire fixation after; see K-wire finger fracture repair
    local anesthetic injection for, 238-239
    tips for, 240-241
    WALANT advantages for, 237
Fingertip
    numbness in, 195
    white, 27
Flexor carpi radialis
    ligament reconstruction and tendon interposition with, 167
    tendon transfer involving, 250
Flexor carpi ulnaris, 250
Flexor digitorum profundus, 193

Flexor digitorum superficialis
    description of, 193
    to flexor pollicis longus tendon
        transfer, 228
    swan neck transfer of, 251
Flexor pollicis longus
    flexor digitorum superficialis tendon
        transfer to, 228
    laceration of, 249
    repair of, 251
Flexor sheath ganglion surgery, 155-156
Flexor tendon repair
    of finger
        anesthesiologist participation in,
            192
        digital extension-flexion test after,
            195
        full active fist testing after, 197
        intraoperative testing, 187
        local anesthetic injection for, 190-
            192
        patient education during, 188
        postoperative regimen for, 196-197
        rectangular flap incisions in, 191
        sheathotomy, 194
        superficialis repair, 189
        tenolysis rates, 187-188
        tips for, 193-195
        WALANT advantages for, 187-189
    of forearm
        anesthesiologist participation in,
            207
        local anesthetic injection for, 207
        tips for, 208
        WALANT advantages for, 205
    of hand
        anesthesiologist participation in,
            202
        extension-flexion test after, 202
        incisions for, 200
        local anesthetic injection for, 200-
            202
        tips for, 202
        WALANT advantages for, 199
    hand therapy in, 113-114
    talking with patients during, 60
    tenolysis rate reduction, 187-188
Forearm
    dorsal, 4
    extensor tendon repair of
        anesthesiologist participation in,
            219
        incisions for, 217

        local anesthetic injection for, 217-
            218
        tips for, 219
        WALANT advantages for, 217
    flexor tendon repair of
        anesthesiologist participation in, 207
        local anesthetic injection for, 207
        tips for, 208
        WALANT advantages for, 205
    radial, 5
    ulnar, 5
    volar, 4
Forearm fascia, 132
Full sterility
    definition of, 69
    field sterility versus, 69-72

G
General anesthesia
    in children, 67
    WALANT and, 100
Germann, Günter, 102
Governments, 78

H
Hand
    flexor tendon repair of; see Flexor
        tendon repair, of hand
    palmaris longus tendon graft for
        rupture of fourth and fifth
        extensor of, 251
    wound to, cleaning of, 249
Hand surgery, complex reconstructions
    in, 249-250
Hand therapists, 111-115
Hemostasis, epinephrine for, 20, 23-24,
    50, 105
Homodigital island flap, 250
Hong Kong, 33
Hospitals
    cost reductions for, 77-78
    profitability for, 77-78

I
Incision
    bleeding from, 136
    after injections, 104
    pain caused by, 62
    redness around, 63
Infants, 65-67
Infection
    hands, 34
    wound, 63, 70-72

Injections, local anesthetics
  0.5 ml with perpendicular needle just
    under dermis, 40-41
  for Bennett fracture, 244
  "blow slow before you go" rule for,
    41-42
  blunt cannulas for, 45-46, 218, 229
  carpal tunnel decompression/release
    using, 130-133
  in children, 65-67
  common mistakes in, 43
  cubital tunnel decompression using,
    138-139
  De Quervain release using, 149-150
  details of, 44
  Dupuytren's contracture surgery
    using, 152-153
  extensor tendon repairs using
    forearm, 217-218
    hand, 214-215
  fainting during, 51-52, 57
  feedback from patient about, 43
  finger amputation using, 125-128
  finger fracture reduction using, 238-
    239
  flexor sheath ganglion surgery using,
    155-156
  flexor tendon repairs using
    finger, 190-192
    hand, 200-202
  incision after, 104
  K-wire finger fracture repair using,
    239
  lacerated nerve repair using, 233-235
  median nerve release at elbow using,
    142-143
  metacarpal fracture reduction and
    internal fixation using, 244-245
  needle should never get ahead of
    local anesthetic, 41-42
  pain-free, rules for, 37-44
  patient positioning during, 52
  proximal interphalangeal joint
    arthroplasty using, 162-163
  reinserting needles within 1 cm of
    blanched/unblanched border, 43
  sensory noise in area of, 38-39, 201
  sharp needles for, 44
  skin cancer excision using, 158-159
  small-bore 27- or 30-gauge needles
    for, 38, 126, 191
  talking with patients during, 61
  tenolysis using, 222-223
  thumb metacarpophalangeal joint
    fusion using, 172
  timing of, 83, 108
  trapeziectomy using, 166-168
  trigger finger surgery using, 146-147
  ulnar collateral ligament repair using,
    172
  vasovagal attack secondary to, 51-52
  volume recommendations, 44
  wrist arthroscopy using, 180-181
Insulin syringe, 33
Insurance companies
  cost reductions for, 78
  profitability for, 78
  WALANT buy-in by, 82
Internal fixation
  of finger fracture; see K-wire finger
    fracture repair
  of metacarpal fracture
    local anesthetic injection for, 244-
    245
    tips for, 246
    WALANT advantages for, 243
Intralipid, 50
Island flap, homodigital, 250

K

Kerrigan, Carolyn, 91-92, 130
Kleinert rubber bands, 188
K-wire finger fracture repair
  field sterility for, 71
  hand therapy in, 114-115
  local anesthetic injection for, 239
  minor procedure rooms for, 120
  talking with patients during, 60
  tips for, 240
  WALANT advantages for, 237

L

Lacerated nerve repair
  digital nerve, 233
  local anesthetic injection for, 233-235
  median nerve, 234-235
  tips for, 235-236
  WALANT advantages for, 233
Lacertus syndrome
  characteristics of, 141
  diagnosis of, 141
  local anesthetic injection for, 142-143
  median nerve release at elbow for,
    141-144
  tips for, 144
Liability, 86

Lidocaine
  adverse reactions to, 50
  anaphylaxis, 49
  history of, 49
  onset of anesthesia with, 30
  safety of, 17, 49-50
  seizures caused by, 50
Lidocaine (1%) with 1:100,000 epineph-
    rine
  buffering of, with 10:1 8.4% sodium
      bicarbonate, 37-38, 138
  carpal tunnel release using, 130-131,
      133
  De Quervain release using, 149
  dilution of, 32
  dosage of, 31-32
  Dupuytren's contracture surgery
      using, 152
  extensor tendon repairs using
    finger, 210
    forearm, 217
    hand, 214
  finger fracture repair using, 238
  flexor sheath ganglion surgery using,
      155
  flexor tendon repairs using
    finger, 190-191
    forearm, 206
    hand, 200-201
  in infants, 66
  lacerated nerve repair using, 233-235
  lacertus tunnel release using, 142
  lipoma excision using, 160
  median nerve laceration repair using,
      234
  metacarpal fracture reduction and
      internal fixation using, 244
  open triangular fibrocartilage
      complex repair using, 184-185
  pH of, 37
  proximal interphalangeal joint
      applications of
    arthroplasty, 162
    fusion, 175
  proximal phalanx injection of, 27
  ray amputation using, 127
  skin cancer excision using, 158
  tendon transfers using, 228-229
  tenolysis using, 222-223
  thumb metacarpophalangeal joint
      fusion using, 172
  trapeziectomy using, 166, 168
  trigger finger surgery using, 146
  trigger thumb surgery using, 146
  ulnar collateral ligament repair using,
      172
  vasoconstriction duration with, 32
  wrist arthroplasty using, 180
Lidocaine with epinephrine; see also Epi-
    nephrine
  0.5% with 1:200,000 epinephrine, 132,
      228, 239
  1% with 1:100,000 epinephrine; see
      Lidocaine (1%) with 1:100,000
      epinephrine
  1% with 1:200,000 epinephrine, 33,
      138
  adverse reactions to, 50
  duration of anesthesia with, 51, 104
  maximal dose of, 49
  numbness duration with, 104
  safety of, 49-50, 83
  talking with patients during injection
      of, 61
Ligament reconstruction and tendon in-
    terposition, 165, 167
Lipid emulsion therapy, 50
Lipoma excision, 160
Litigation, 77
Local anesthesia
  hospital operating rooms for, 90
  perspectives on, 34-35, 92-93
  sedation versus, 89
  tumescent; see Tumescent local
      anesthesia
Local anesthetics
  bupivacaine, 50-51
  diffusion of
    in middorsal hand, 9, 126-127
    in midline dorsal forearm, 4
    in midline dorsal wrist, 6
    in midline radial forearm, 5
    in midline radial wrist, 7
    in midline ulnar forearm, 5
    in midline ulnar wrist, 8
    in midline volar forearm, 4
    in midline volar wrist, 6
    in midpalmar hand, 8, 125, 127,
        162, 175
    natural barriers to, 34
    in thumb midmetacarpal dorsal, 10
    in thumb midmetacarpal volar, 10
    in ulnar hand, 9
  injection of
    0.5 ml with perpendicular needle
        just under dermis, 40-41

Bennett fracture surgery using, 244
"blow slow before you go" rule for, 41-42
blunt cannulas for, 45-46, 218, 229
carpal tunnel decompression/ release using, 130-133
in children, 65-67
common mistakes in, 43
De Quervain release using, 149-150
details of, 44
Dupuytren's contracture surgery using, 152-153
extensor tendon repair of forearm using, 217-218
extensor tendon repair of hand using, 214-215
fainting during, 51-52, 57
feedback from patient about, 43
finger amputation using, 125-128
finger fracture reduction using, 238-239
flexor sheath ganglion surgery using, 155-156
flexor tendon repair of finger using, 190-192
flexor tendon repair of hand using, 200-202
incision after, 104
K-wire finger fracture repair using, 239
lacerated nerve repair using, 233-235
median nerve release at elbow using, 142-143
metacarpal fracture reduction and internal fixation using, 244-245
needle should never get ahead of local anesthetic, 41-42
or cubital tunnel decompression using, 138-139
pain-free, rules for, 37-44
patient positioning during, 52
proximal interphalangeal joint arthroplasty using, 162-163
reinserting needles within 1 cm of blanched/unblanched border, 43
sensory noise in area of, 38-39, 201
sharp needles for, 44
skin cancer excision using, 158-159
small-bore 27- or 30-gauge needles for, 38, 126, 191
talking with patients during, 61
tenolysis using, 222-223

thumb metacarpophalangeal joint fusion using, 172
timing of, 83, 108
trapeziectomy using, 166-168
trigger finger surgery using, 146-147
ulnar collateral ligament repair using, 172
vasovagal attack secondary to, 51-52
volume recommendations, 44
wrist arthroscopy using, 180-181
lidocaine; see Lidocaine
longer-lasting, 50-51
refrigeration of, 38
ropivacaine, 50
volume recommendations for, 44
Lymphedema, 94

M
MacFarlane, Bobby, 23
Median nerve
anesthetic block of, 129
carpal tunnel decompression of; see Carpal tunnel decompression/ release
laceration repair of, local anesthetic injection for, 234-235
release of, at elbow
anesthesiologist participation in, 143
local anesthetic injection for, 142-143
tips for, 144
WALANT advantages for, 141-142
Merritt splint, 209, 213
Metacarpal fracture reduction and internal fixation
local anesthetic injection for, 244-245
WALANT advantages for, 243
Metaphalangeal fractures, 241
Middorsal hand, local anesthetic diffusion pattern in, 9, 126-127
Midline dorsal forearm, local anesthetic diffusion pattern in, 4
Midline dorsal wrist, local anesthetic diffusion pattern in, 6
Midline radial forearm, local anesthetic diffusion pattern in, 5
Midline radial wrist, local anesthetic diffusion pattern in, 7
Midline ulnar forearm, local anesthetic diffusion pattern in, 5

Midline ulnar wrist, local anesthetic diffusion pattern in, 8
Midline volar forearm, local anesthetic diffusion pattern in, 4
Midline volar wrist, local anesthetic diffusion pattern in, 6
Midpalmar hand, local anesthetic diffusion pattern in, 8, 125, 127, 162, 175
Minor procedure rooms
    cleaning of, 118
    equipment in, 118-120
    facilities near, 121
    field sterility in, 119
    hand trauma, 120-121
    personnel, 118
    physical space of, 117-118
    procedures not performed in, 121
    reception area, 117
    surgical equipment in, 118-120
Mohs surgery, 70
Monoamine oxidase, 51
Motion extension splint, 209, 213, 219

N

Needles
    "blow slow before you go" rule for, 41-42
    blunt cannulas versus, 45
    perpendicular, injection of 0.5 ml just under dermis using, 40-41
    reinserting of, within 1 cm of blanched/unblanched border, 43
    for sedation versus WALANT, 56
    20-gauge, 56
    27- or 30-gauge, for local anesthetic injections, 38, 56, 126, 147, 150, 156, 172, 191
Nelson, David L., 100
Nerve, lacerated; see Lacerated nerve repair
Neurapraxia, ischemic, 27
Nurses, 20
    barriers to WALANT by, 85-86
    liability concerns of, 86
    WALANT buy-in by, 79-81
    working with, 91

O

Open carpal tunnel decompression/release
    local anesthetic injection for, 130-132
    tips for, 134-135

Open triangular fibrocartilage complex repair
    anesthesiologist participation in, 185
    local anesthetic injection for, 184-185
    tips for, 186
    WALANT advantages for, 183
Operating rooms
    time out in, 84
    WALANT procedures in, 72

P

Pain
    fear of, 84-85
    feeling of, after injection, 85
    management of, 89
    types of, 62
Palmar/dorsal borders, local anesthetic diffusion affected by, 34
Palmaris longus tendon graft, 251
Paresthesia, 29, 44
Patient(s)
    anxious, 52, 55
    barriers to WALANT by, 84-85
    calming of, 86
    compliance by, 20
    cost decreases for, 75-76
    expectations of, 55
    fainting by, during injection, 51-52
    fears of, 84-85
    hand therapists for, 112-113
    monitoring of, 121
    satisfaction of, 95, 102
    scheduling of, 107-108
    talking with; see also Patient education
        during carpal tunnel release, 62-63
        during consultation, 55-57
        during local anesthetic injection, 61
        during surgery, 59-60, 87
        on day of surgery, 57-58
    WALANT benefits for, 18-19, 56, 75-76, 100-101
Patient education; see also Patient(s), talking with
    about procedure, 59-60
    during flexor tendon repair of finger, 188
    during trigger finger surgery, 147-148
    intraoperative, 76
Payers
    cost reductions for, 78
    WALANT buy-in by, 79-82
Pediatrics, 65-67

Phentolamine, 24-27, 50, 83
Pilot study, 80
Postoperative period
     after carpal tunnel release, 62-63
     after flexor tendon repair of finger,
          196-197
     WALANT benefits, 18, 57
Preoperative testing, 76
Procaine, 25
Profitability, 77-78
Propofol, 31, 81, 86, 88, 104, 135, 143,
          163, 168, 173, 176, 182, 185, 192,
          202, 207, 211, 215, 219, 224, 230
Proximal interphalangeal joint (PIP)
     arthroplasty of
          anesthesiologist participation in,
               163
          local anesthetic injection for, 162-
               163
          tips for, 163
          WALANT advantages for, 161
     comminuted fracture of, 241
     dorsal fracture dislocations of, 240
     fusion of
          anesthesiologist participation in,
               176
          local anesthetic injection for, 175-
               176
          tips for, 177
          WALANT advantages for, 175
Proximal phalanx
     dorsal thumb, anesthetic block of, 13
     subcutaneous midline, with lidocaine
          and epinephrine, 11

R
Ray amputation
     local anesthetic injection for, 125-128
     tips and tricks for, 128
     WALANT advantages for, 125
Regitine; see Phentolamine
Reimbursement, 87, 92, 96
Residents
     education of, 61
     WALANT participation by, 87-88
Revenue, for surgeons, 76, 87
Ropivacaine, 50

S
Safety checklists, 90
Sauerbier, Michael, 221
Scars, 34, 44
Scheduling of patients, 107-108

Sedation
     advantages of not using, 129
     in anxious patients, 52
     costs associated with, 77
     culture regarding need for, in surgery,
          90
     lack of need for, 21
     local anesthesia versus, 89
     patient satisfaction and, 90
Seizures, lidocaine-induced, 50
Senn retractors, 103, 118
Sensory noise, 38-39, 201
Sheathotomy, 194
Shoemaker, Pat, 23
Single subcutaneous injection in the
          proximal phalanx with lidocaine
          and epinephrine (SIMPLE)
     with dorsal block augmentation, 12
     for finger amputation, 127
     illustration of, 11
     thumb block, 11
     two dorsal injection block versus, 46-
          47
Skin
     creases in, local anesthetic diffusion
          affected by, 34, 44
     sensory noise in, 39
Skin cancer excision
     local anesthetic injection for, 158-159
     patient education during, 157
     tips for, 159-160
     WALANT advantages for, 157-158
Sodium bicarbonate (10:1 8.4%), for
          buffering of 1% lidocaine with
          1:100,000 epinephrine, 37-38,
          138
Soft tissue excisions
     lipomas, 160
     skin cancer, 157-160
"Space-suit" operating room sterility, 71
"Spaghetti wrist" injury, 205
Stakeholders, 79-80
Sterility; see Field sterility; Full sterility
Students, 87-88
Surgeons
     anesthesiologist and, 86
     barriers to WALANT by, 86-88
     case studies of, 91-97
     cost benefits for, 76-78
     reimbursement concerns of, 87, 92
     revenue for, 76, 87
     wide awake hand surgery benefits for,
          20-21

Swan neck transfer, of flexor digitorum superficialis, 251
Syringe, stabilization of, 39
Szabo, Robert, 227

T

Tendon reconstruction, 56
Tendon transfers
    anesthesiologist participation in, 230
    extensor indicis to extensor pollicis longus, 227-228
    flexor carpi radialis and flexor carpi ulnaris, 250
    flexor digitorum superficialis to flexor pollicis longus, 228
    local anesthetic injection for, 228-229
    tension on, 227
    tips for, 230-231
    WALANT advantages for, 227
Tenolysis
    anesthesiologist participation in, 224
    local anesthetic injection for, 222-223
    patient education during, 225
    postoperative instructions, 224
    talking with patient during, 221-222
    tips for, 224-225
    WALANT advantages for, 221-222
30-gauge needles, for local anesthetic injection, 38
Thumb
    anesthetic block of, single subcutaneous injection in the proximal phalanx with lidocaine and epinephrine for, 12
    basal joint arthritis of, trapeziectomy for; see Trapeziectomy
    extension restoration in, after subtotal amputation, 250
    extensor pollicis longus tendon of, 230
    midmetacarpal dorsal, 10
    midmetacarpal volar, 10
    trigger; see Trigger finger surgery
Thumb metacarpophalangeal joint fusion
    anesthesiologist participation in, 173
    local anesthetic injection for, 172
    tips for, 173
    WALANT advantages for, 171
Thumb tip pinch, after adult pollicization, 249
"Top-ups," 30, 44

Tourniquet, 19, 75, 102-103
Trainees, 61
Trapeziectomy
    anesthesiologist participation in, 168
    local anesthetic injection for, 166-168
    tips for, 168-169
    WALANT advantages for, 165-166
Triangular fibrocartilage complex repair, open
    anesthesiologist participation in, 185
    local anesthetic injection for, 184-185
    tips for, 186
    WALANT advantages for, 183
Trigger finger surgery
    in children, 67
    field sterility for, 70
    local anesthetic injection for, 146-147
    patient education during, 147-148
    tips for, 147-148
    WALANT advantages for, 145-146
    wide awake hand surgery benefits for, 21
Tumescent local anesthesia
    characteristics of, 29
    definition of, 29
    in general anesthesia patients, 29
    injection rules for, 30-31, 44
    for skin cancer excision, 157
    "top-ups," 30
    volume recommendations, 30
27-gauge needles, for local anesthetic injection, 38, 56, 126, 147, 150, 156, 172
Two dorsal injection block, single subcutaneous injection in the proximal phalanx with lidocaine and epinephrine (SIMPLE) block versus, 46-47

U

Ulnar collateral ligament repair
    anesthesiologist participation in, 173
    local anesthetic injection for, 172
    tips for, 173
    WALANT advantages for, 171
Ulnar hand, local anesthetic diffusion pattern in, 9

V

Van Demark, Robert, Jr., 94-97, 100-101
Vasovagal attack, 51-52

W
WALANT
    advantages of, 18-21, 101; *see also specific procedure, WALANT advantages for*
    contraindications for, 103
    description of, 17
    duration of, 57
    general anesthesia and, 100
    getting started, 99-101
    indications for, 93-94, 102-103
    patient benefits from, 18-19
    postoperative recovery from, 18, 57
    safety of, 19, 56, 95
    surgeon benefits from, 20-21
    talking with patients, 55-60
Weilby suspension, 169
White fingertip, 27
Wong, Jason, 102-103, 221, 250

Wound
    care of, after carpal tunnel release, 62
    cleaning of, 249
    infection of, 63, 70-72
Wrist, local anesthetic diffusion patterns in
    dorsal, 6
    radial, 7
    ulnar, 8
    volar, 6
Wrist arthroscopy
    anesthesiologist participation in, 182
    dry, 179
    local anesthetic injection for, 180-181
    tips for, 181-182
    WALANT advantages for, 179
Wrist injections
    concerns about, 35
    for wrist arthroscopy, 180-181
Wrist vein grafts, for finger revascularization, 250